W9-BGP-657

Jeffrey T. Huber, PhD
Kris Riddlesperger, MS, CNS, RN

Eating Positive
A Nutrition Guide and Recipe Book for People with HIV/AIDS

Pre-publication
REVIEWS,
COMMENTARIES,
EVALUATIONS . . .

"**E**ating Positive: A Nutrition Guide and Recipe Book for People with HIV/AIDS is the first book that I have seen that considers the sometimes complicated nutritional needs and challenges of people who are HIV positive. I have tried several of the recipes and give high accolades to both the culinary appeal and ease of preparation of these recipes. Both olfactory and taste appeal and preparation are very important to people who have reduced appetites and energy. The directions are clear and easy to follow, but at the same time, leave room for an individual's creativity. For the recipes that I tried more than once, I reduced the fat content with no adverse effect on the result and was able to present the same meal for friends with differing nutritional requirements.

As a nurse, it is enlightening to finally see the mystery removed from the 'clear liquid' and the 'full liquid' diets. So many times professional health care providers give these orders without adequate direction as to what constitutes the special diet. This type of information, presented in this format, provides many wonderful options for increased caloric and nutritional requirements to my population of concern. Kudos!!"

Sarah C. Fogel, MSN, RN, ACRN
Assistant Professor
of Practicing Nursing,
Vanderbilt University Medical Center,
Nashville, TN

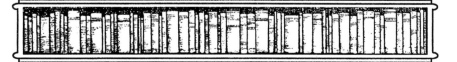

"*E*ating Positive is an excellent resource for people living with HIV/AIDS, especially for those who enjoy experimenting a little in the kitchen. Divided into sections by diet type (clear liquid, full liquid, lactose-free, high-fiber, high-protein/high-calorie, etc.), each segment has a short introduction explaining the purpose of that type of diet. One can tell that the authors know what they're talking about, but they let you know about the nutritional part in folksy, day-to-day language, not in the scientific jargon you so often hear.

Then come the fun recipes. Readers will recognize old favorites like Four-Bean Salad, but will be intrigued by the likes of 24-Hour Wine and Cheese Omelet, Chicken Breasts with Grapes, and One-Eyed Egyptians (this, in 'Bland Diets,' no less!). There is a nice range of complexity (in terms of time, energy, and number of ingredients) as well as diversity in the degree of taste sophistication (from comfort-level Rice Pudding to Watercress Soup.)

Each recipe has been carefully analyzed for nutrient values: total calories and grams of protein, carbohydrates, and fat. This information is an indispensable feature for those conscientiously watching nutrients in their diets.

This is a useful and caring collaboration between a nurse/nutritionist and a PhD/gourmet."

Alison Moreland, RN, MS, FNP
Instructor,
Community Health Nursing,
Texas Christian University,
Fort Worth, TX

"**H**aving taken care of a brother with AIDS, I understand the importance of a good diet. I believe his diet gave me an extra 18 months with him that I otherwise would not have had. However, at times, it was very difficult to maintain creativity in his diet and know what was best for him at the same time. We, as humans, are finally beginning to understand the significance diet has in all of our lives. I applaud the authors of *Eating Positive* for their contribution to people with HIV/AIDS, as well as to those of us who love and care for them."

Michelle M. Wayman, BS
University of North Texas,
Weatherford, TX

Eating Positive
A Nutrition Guide and Recipe Book for People with HIV/AIDS

HAWORTH Medical Information Sources
M. Sandra Wood, MLS, MBA
Senior Editor

New, Recent, and Forthcoming Titles:

How to Find Information About AIDS, 2nd Edition
edited by Jeffrey T. Huber

*CD-ROM Implementation and NeTworking in Health Sciences
Libraries* edited by M. Sandra Wood

User Education in Health Sciences Libraries: A Reader
edited by M. Sandra Wood

*HIV/AIDS Community Information Services: Experiences
in Serving Both At-Risk and HIV-Infected Populations*
by Jeffrey T. Huber

*HIV/AIDS and HIV/AIDS-Related Terminology: A Means
of Organizing the Body of Knowledge* by Jeffrey T. Huber
and Mary L. Gillaspy

*Eating Positive: A Nutrition Guide and Recipe Book for People
with HIV/AIDS* by Jeffrey T. Huber and Kris Riddlesperger

Eating Positive
A Nutrition Guide and Recipe Book for People with HIV/AIDS

Jeffrey T. Huber, PhD
Kris Riddlesperger, MS, CNS, RN

The Haworth Press
New York • London

The Haworth Press, Inc., 10 Alice Street, Binghamton, NY 13904-1580

Cover design by Marylouise E. Doyle.

Library of Congress Cataloging-in-Publication Data

Huber, Jeffrey T.
    Eating positive : a nutrition guide and recipe book for people with HIV/AIDS / Jeffrey T. Huber, Kris Riddlesperger.
        p.   cm.
    Includes index.
    ISBN 0-7890-0103-9 (alk. paper).
    1. AIDS (Disease)—Diet therapy+Recipes. I. Title.
RC607.A26H6952 1998
616.97′920654—dc21

                                                                        97-28285
                                                                            CIP

CONTENTS

ABOUT THE AUTHORS

Jeffrey T. Huber, PhD, is Research Information Scientist in the Active Digital Library of the Eskind Biomedical Library at Venderbilt University in Nashville, Tennessee. He is also Research Assistant Professor in the Division of Biomedical Informatics at Vanderbilt. For two years, Dr. Huber was Assistant Professor at the School of Library and Information Studies at Texas Woman's University in Denton, Texas, where he was also Co-Chair of the University's Task Force on HIV/AIDS. He is the author of *HIV/AIDS Community Information Services: Experiences in Serving Both At-Risk and HIV-Infected Populations* (The Haworth Press, Inc.) and the co-author of *HIV/AIDS and HIV/AIDS-Related Terminology: A Means of Organizing the Body of Knowledge* (The Haworth Press, Inc.). The editor of *How to Find Information About AIDS, Second Edition* and the *Dictionary of AIDS-Related Terminology*, he has written a number of articles concerning AIDS information and has delivered many presentations at national conferences and meetings.

Kris Riddlesperger, MS, RN, is an Assistant Professor of Maternal Child Nursing at Texas Christian University in Fort Worth, Texas. She is currently completing her PhD in nursing at Texas Woman's University in Denton, Texas. Her dissertation research is focused on nursing interventions with health policy and the HIV-positive client. She is a Clinical Nurse Specialist in women's health and has been a practicing nurse for 12 years. She has been teaching at the university level for the past three years.

Acknowledgments

The authors gratefully wish to acknowledge the assistance of Jana K. Kastelhun and Byron Wilson for their assistance in preparing this manuscript.

Introduction

Nutritional support is essential to individuals with HIV/AIDS. Yet proper nutrition is often difficult to maintain due to a variety of conditions and complications associated with the disease and/or with medications commonly prescribed for treatment. This work is designed to facilitate maintenance of nutritional intake based on diet types intended to counteract conditions and complications that foster or exacerbate malnutrition.

This book came into being as a guide for cooking for HIV-positive people when the authors realized they had two unique perspectives on the management of food. Kris enjoys figuring out nutritional balance and finding ways to help people eat when the mechanics of eating may be a problem. Jeffrey has a true appreciation for food and the culinary arts. The two authors were linked through various research interests in HIV and found out that each had contact with a special person with an eating problem with which the other could assist. For Kris, it was a child who needed to increase her nutrition and calorie intake but who found food to be unappealing and not really worth the effort to eat. For Jeffrey, it was a friend who had terrible difficulty with mouth ulcers. Eating food was a mechanical challenge as well as a taste issue. Between the two, they came up with a few interesting recipes and the idea for this book.

This book is to be used as a reference manual for the common types of diets HIV-positive people may find useful or be directed toward by their health care provider. In no way is this a prescriptive manual, rather it is an entry to cooking by diet type designed to explain the diet, list the foods commonly found within the diet, and give guidance through recipes in the combinations of foods available within the diet. This is not a comprehensive book; it is a primer for preparing food for the HIV-positive person experiencing some special dietary problems, and a guide to creating and eating the right food for the right person on the right diet, at the right time in the right form.

The book is organized into three sections. The Introduction serves as an overview of nutritional issues associated with HIV/ AIDS and discusses the intended use of this book. The second section constitutes the bulk of the work in that it includes actual recipes accompanied by their respective nutritional values. Recipes are organized in chapters reflective of specific diet needs. Each chapter begins with a list of recipes included therein followed by a brief introduction describing diet type, benefits, and potential hazards. Diet types may be broadly divided into clear liquid; full liquid; fiber restricted; bananas, rice, applesauce, and tea (B.R.A.T.); lactose-free; high-fiber; bland; and high protein/high calorie. Each type addresses the degree of restriction placed on an individual. Within each diet type, specific recipes are included to account for particular nutritional needs. This is not to say, of course, that recipes associated with a particular diet type may not be appropriate for another diet type. Recipes within each chapter are arranged in order of preparation difficulty beginning with those requiring the least amount of effort and knowledge of food preparation. Nutritional values (i.e., calories, fat, carbohydrates, and protein) are included for each recipe. In general, the number of servings per recipe is derived within the context of the respective diet. In addition, helpful hints, suggestions, and variations are interspersed throughout. The final section is comprised of an index arranged by food groups or recipe type and an alphabetic index. A glossary of terms is also included at the end of the book.

Tips for Eating

There are times when there is the desire to eat but the mouth cannot do it. Perhaps you are having difficulty with oral ulcers, or thrush, or just cannot chew. Here are some ideas to try.

1. If alcohol is allowed in your diet, try swishing out the mouth with whiskey and spitting it out just as you might use a mouthwash. The whiskey will burn (use a test amount first) but then has a numbing effect on the tissues. It is short-term relief but may be enough to help get some food down.

2. Almost anything can be put in a blender. Whether trying to load calories or simply get some vegetables down, if the texture is causing mouth pain or if it is just too hard to chew and swallow, the food can be softened either a lot or a little depending on the need.

3. Straws are a great way to bypass mouth pain and get the nutrition into the person, and they can be fun, too.

4. Check the temperature of the food. While our grandmothers taught us to serve it "piping hot" that may cause pain in a tender mouth, as might freezing cold. Remember getting your lips stuck on an icicle as a child? Well, that is to be avoided when there is trouble with mouth ulcers, so perhaps the popsicle should be crushed up and slurped or spooned.

5. If the jaw muscles are weak or painful, massaging them before eating could be helpful in the chewing process. Sometimes it is even helpful to apply a soft heating pad to the jaw area (not too hot; you do not want to burn yourself) right before mealtime.

Bon Appetite!

Clear Liquid Diet

Recipes

Apple Cooler
Iced Tea
Lemonade
Grape Shrub
Instant Russian Tea
Hot Spiced Cider

* * *

Clear liquids are just that, clear. This diet has a water base and is meant to assist in avoiding dehydration when one cannot eat or drink a regular diet. This diet is not nutritionally balanced alone and would not be used for long periods of time unless ordered by the health care provider. (Consult your primary health care provider for anything longer than 24 to 48 hours.) One would select this diet when there is difficulty eating due to fever, nausea, vomiting, diarrhea, or mouth pain. This diet assists in slowing the intestine and avoiding irritating foods and spices. It can be soothing to the mouth, because there are no sharp corners or rubbing as occurs when chewing food. It is also a good way to introduce food back to an individual after a prolonged period without food, such as the time following certain surgical procedures. This diet works best when the liquids are offered in small amounts frequently throughout the day; for example, a cup of broth and a scoop of gelatin, rather than a quart of broth at one sitting. It also is helpful to pander to the individual's tastes as much as possible. Frankly, a clear liquid diet can get boring rapidly, so anything to encourage it is helpful. We recommend using as many different foods from the list as possible. This also helps to balance the available nutrition in the diet. Other tips to keep in mind with this diet are, first, caffeine in large quantities may be overstimulating, especially to the bowel; and second, carbonated drinks may cause a "gassy" feeling.

Below are examples of the foodstuffs included in this diet:

- water
- strained, clear fruit juice
- flavored and unflavored gelatin
- low fat and fat free broths
- popsicles
- fruit ices
- sugar

- hard candy
- coffee
- tea
- clear soda
- nondairy sherbet
- honey
- syrup

SUGGESTIONS

- Substitute Pedialyte or Infalyte for water to help replenish electrolytes depleted by vomiting or diarrhea.
- Add a slice of lemon, lime, or orange to flavor a glass of water. (Just a slice, though! Not a half or whole.)

SAMPLE RECIPES

Apple Cooler

Combine equal parts apple juice and ginger ale. Pour over ice cubes.

Nutrient Value per Serving (per cup): 99.76 calories, 0.07g protein, 25.12g carbohydrates, 0.14g fat

Variation: Substitute grape juice for apple juice.

Iced Tea

1 1/2 cups water
6 tea bags
1/2 cup sugar

Bring water to boil in a small saucepan. Add tea bags. Cover and remove from heat. Allow tea bags to steep for 3 to 5 minutes. Pour tea into 2-quart pitcher, leaving tea bags in saucepan. Refill saucepan with cold water, squeezing tea bags to release additional flavor. Add to pitcher. Repeat to fill pitcher. Stir in sugar. Refrigerate.

Nutrient Value per Serving (makes 3 servings): 129 calories, 0g protein, 33.3g carbohydrates, 0g fat

Lemonade

fresh lemons
1 cup sugar
1 cup cold water

Squeeze enough lemons to yield 1 cup lemon juice. Dissolve sugar in lemon juice and water. Pour into 2-quart pitcher. Add enough cold water to fill pitcher. Float additional lemon slices in lemonade. Serve in glasses over ice.

Nutrient Value per Serving (makes 4 servings): 210.32 calories, 0.65g protein, 55.36g carbohydrates, 0.18g fat

Variation: Mix equal parts of lemonade and cranberry juice.

Grape Shrub

1 cup lemon nondairy sherbet
1/4 cup grape juice

Place sherbet in a dish. Top with juice.

Nutrient Value per Serving (makes 1 serving): 304.92 calories, 2.48g protein, 68.16g carbohydrates, 3.91g fat

Variation: Substitute pineapple nondairy sherbet and orange juice.

Instant Russian Tea

1 cup instant tea with lemon and sugar
11-ounce jar Tang
1 teaspoon sugar
1 teaspoon ground cloves
1 large package presweetened powdered lemonade

Mix all ingredients well. Store in an airtight container.

For 1 cup of tea, add boiling water to 2½ teaspoons of powdered mixture and serve.

Nutrient Value per Serving (per teaspoon): 10.22 calories, 0g protein, 2.63g carbohydrates, 0g fat

Hot Spiced Cider

1 gallon apple cider
1 4-ounce can frozen orange juice concentrate
1 3-ounce can frozen cranberry juice
1/4 teaspoon ground allspice
1/4 teaspoon ground cloves
2 drops cassia oil (cinnamon)

Mix ingredients well, heat, and serve in mugs or cups.

Nutrient Value per Serving (per cup): 61.72 calories, 0.10g protein, 15.36g carbohydrates, 0.14g fat

Notes

Full Liquid Diet

Recipes

Fortified Milk
Orange Cow
Easy Egg-Drop Soup
Cherry Dessert
Cottage Cheese Jello Salad
Orange Jello Salad
Lime Jello Salad

Tropical Frozen Delight
Custard
Fluffy Peach Jello
Cheese Soup
Cream of Carrot Soup
Creamy Pumpkin Soup
Cheese Souffle

*   *   *

Unlike the Clear Liquid Diet, the Full Liquid Diet is much more nutritionally balanced and can, with the planning and advising of a nutritional counselor, meet full nutritional needs over a long period of time. This diet can also be a stepping-stone or a transition between the clear liquid diet and the low-fiber diet as a person is working to return to a more generalized diet. The consistency of the food makes this a good option for people with mouth pain and difficulty chewing and it, too, is easy on the digestive system (assuming there is no lactose intolerance).

Foods on this diet include all those on the clear liquid diet list as well as those listed below. A rule of thumb for this diet is that it may include any food which is a liquid at body temperature and does not contain fruit, nuts, seeds, raw eggs, or bread.

Foodstuffs included in this diet consist of all those in the clear liquid regimen plus those in the following list:

- milk/milk-based products
- soda
- coffee
- tea
- instant drink mixes of any kind
- strained juices
- refined cooked cereals
- strained whole grains
- protein powders
- puddings
- gelatin (Jello)
- custards
- pumpkin
- ice cream
- marshmallow
- frozen yogurt
- plain, vanilla, or lemon yogurt
- eggs cooked to liquid
- egg substitutes
- eggnogs
- brewer's yeast
- cinnamon
- nutmeg
- flavorings
- syrups
- nectars
- cornstarch
- margarine
- butter
- cream soups with vegetable, meats, or potatoes
- finely homogenized meat
- purees

ABSOLUTELY NO:

- breads
- "raw" cereals
- nuts
- fruits
- seeds
- raw eggs
- solids

SAMPLE RECIPES

Fortified Milk

1 quart milk
1 cup instant nonfat dry milk
Pour milk into deep bowl. Add dry milk and beat slowly with a beater or whisk until milk is dissolved. Refrigerate.

Nutrient Value per Serving (makes 4 servings): 210.68 calories, 14.02g protein, 20.27g carbohydrates, 8.3g fat

Orange Cow

3 scoops vanilla ice cream
3/4 to 1 cup orange juice

Place ice cream and juice in blender or drink mixer. Blend until smooth. (Adjust the amount of juice for desired thickness.)

Nutrient Value per Serving (makes 2 servings): 323.13 calories, 5.53g protein, 44.29g carbohydrates, 14.88g fat

Easy Egg Drop Soup

2 cups chicken broth
1 egg
salt and pepper to taste

Bring chicken broth to boil in a heavy saucepan. Reduce heat to a simmer. Beat egg in a bowl until well blended. Slowly pour the beaten egg over the back of a fork into the simmering chicken broth. (Avoid dropping the egg into the broth to keep it from clumping.) Stir gently for a minute. Remove from heat. Salt and pepper to taste. Serve immediately.

Nutrient Value per Serving (makes 2 servings): 59.21 calories, 4.47g protein, 1.75g carbohydrates, 3.6g fat

Cherry Dessert

1 8-ounce carton Cool Whip
1 can Eagle Brand condensed milk
1 can cherry pie filling

Line loaf pan with foil. Mix ingredients well. Pour mixture into lined loaf pan and freeze overnight. Invert pan and remove foil. Slice dessert and serve. Keep frozen.

Nutrient Value per Serving (makes 4 servings): 263.43 calories, 6.05g protein, 40.11g carbohydrates, 9.57g fat

Cottage Cheese Jello Salad

1 8-ounce carton cottage cheese (small curd)
1 8-ounce carton Cool Whip
1 3-ounce package Jello

Fold Cool Whip into cottage cheese. Sprinkle dry Jello over mixture and mix well. Refrigerate and chill. Stir once or twice while mixture chills in refrigerator.

Nutrient Value per Serving (makes 4 servings): 304.75 calories, 29.18g protein, 23.93g carbohydrates, 12.40g fat

Orange Jello Salad

1 6-ounce package orange Jello
2 cups hot water
1 pint orange sherbet

Dissolve Jello in hot water. Stir in softened sherbet. Chill and serve.

Nutrient Value per Serving (makes 4 servings): 274.75 calories, 3.94g protein, 62.94g carbohydrates, 1.93g fat

Variation: Substitute other Jello flavors and complementary sherbets.

Lime Jello Salad

1 3-ounce package lime Jello
1/2 cup sugar
1 1/2 cups hot water
1 cup small marshmallows
1 8-ounce package cream cheese
1 cup Cool Whip

Dissolve Jello, sugar, and marshmallows in hot water. Stir until all are dissolved. Place in refrigerator and chill until thickened. Stir in softened cream cheese. Fold in Cool Whip. Chill and serve.

Nutrient Value per Serving (makes 2 servings): 934.50 calories, 11.51g protein, 146.43g carbohydrates, 15.48g fat

Tropical Frozen Delight

1 6-ounce can frozen orange juice
1 large can Carnation evaporated milk (1 2/3 cup)
1/4 cup lemon juice
1/2 cup sugar

Soften frozen orange juice. Pour Carnation evaporated milk into flat dish and freeze until ice crystals form (approximately 30 minutes). Pour crystalized Carnation into large bowl and whip with an egg beater until stiff (approximately 2 minutes). Add lemon juice and continue beating until very stiff (2 to 3 minutes). Mix sugar and softened orange juice into Carnation mixture with wooden spoon. Pour into two loaf pans or one 9 x 13-inch baking dish and freeze overnight.

Nutrient Value per Serving (makes 2 servings): 834.11 calories, 16.42g protein, 163.38g carbohydrates, 15.53g fat

Custard

1 cup sugar
1 dash salt
5 tablespoons flour
3 egg yolks
2 1/2 cups milk
1 teaspoon butter
1 teaspoon vanilla

Add flour, sugar, and salt. Beat egg yolks and add milk slowly to beaten yolks. Add egg and milk mixture to flour mixture. Add butter. Cook slowly over medium low heat stirring constantly until mixture thickens. Remove from heat. Cool and add vanilla. Refrigerate.

Nutrient Value per Serving (makes 4 servings): 372.46 calories, 8.58g protein, 63.64g carbohydrates, 9.82g fat

Fluffy Peach Jello

1 cup canned peaches with syrup
1 package peach Jello
1 cup boiling water

Place peaches with syrup in blender or food processor. Puree. Pour pureed peaches into measuring cup and add enough syrup or water to make one cup. Dissolve Jello in boiling water. Pour into a deep bowl. Add peach puree. Blend completely. Refrigerate until Jello thickens but is not firm. Remove from refrigerator and whip the Jello until fluffy and doubled in volume. Refrigerate until firm.

Nutrient Value per Serving (makes 2 servings): 144.90 calories, 1.60g protein, 37.38g carbohydrates, 0.13g fat

Variation: Substitute other fruits and complementary Jello flavors.

Cheese Soup

4 tablespoons butter
4 cups heavy cream
2 cloves garlic
4 cups grated cheddar cheese
4 egg yolks

Mince garlic. Beat egg yolks and combine with 1 cup of cream. Place butter in heavy saucepan. Add garlic and sauté over medium heat until garlic is wilted. Reduce heat to medium to low. Add 3 cups of cream and cheese, stirring constantly. Cook until cheese is melted. Stir in egg yolk mixture. Cook until heated through, but do not boil.

Nutrient Value per Serving (makes 4 servings): 1,439.97 calories, 36.05g protein, 8.93g carbohydrates, 142.12g fat

Cream of Carrot Soup

2 tablespoons margarine
6 large carrots
6 green onions (including green stalks)
4 cups chicken broth
1 cup heavy cream
salt and pepper
bay leaf

Chop carrots and green onions. Melt margarine in large saucepan. Add chopped carrots and green onions. Stir. Add chicken broth and bay leaf. Bring to a boil. Reduce heat. Cover and simmer approximately 45 minutes or until carrots are tender. Remove bay leaf. Transfer mixture to a blender or food processor and puree (in batches if necessary). Be sure mixture is smooth. Return mixture to saucepan. Add cream. Salt and pepper to taste. Stir over low heat until heated through (do not boil). Serve.

Nutrient Value per Serving (makes 4 servings): 330 calories, 4.1g protein, 15.46g carbohydrates, 28.99g fat

Creamy Pumpkin Soup

3 tablespoons margarine
1 medium onion, chopped
1 tablespoon flour
1 teaspoon salt
1/8 teaspoon ground ginger
1/8 teaspoon freshly grated nutmeg
1/8 teaspoon ground cloves
bay leaf
4 cups chicken broth
1 14-ounce can pumpkin
1 cup heavy cream

Melt margarine in large saucepan over medium heat. Add chopped onion and sauté until soft and wilted. Blend in flour, salt, ginger, nutmeg, and cloves. Stirring constantly, cook 2 to 3 minutes. Add the chicken broth and pumpkin. Mix well. Add bay leaf. Cover and simmer approximately 30 minutes. Remove bay leaf. Transfer mixture to a blender or food processor and puree (in batches if necessary). Be sure mixture is smooth. Return mixture to saucepan. Add cream. Stir over low heat until heated through (do not boil). Serve.

Nutrient Value per Serving (makes 4 servings): 351.18 calories, 4.20g protein, 14.45g carbohydrates, 31.90g fat

Cheese Soufflé

3 1/2 tablespoons butter
4 1/2 tablespoons flour
1 1/2 cups hot milk
1/2 teaspoon salt
1/8 teaspoon pepper
Pinch ground nutmeg
6 egg yolks
8 egg whites, room temperature
1/2 teaspoon cream of tartar
Pinch of salt
4 ounces (1 cup pressed down) coarsely grated Swiss cheese or mixture of Swiss and Parmesan
1 tablespoon butter for dish
2 tablespoons grated Swiss for topping

Rub soufflé dish with butter. Melt butter in saucepan. Blend in flour. Stir over medium heat to cook. Remove from heat. Blend in hot milk all at once, whisking vigorously. Add salt, pepper, nutmeg, and return to heat. Stir with whisk and boil 1 minute. Sauce will be very thick. Remove from heat. Whisk in yolks one at a time. Beat 8 egg whites on low speed with mixer to foaming. Add cream of tartar and salt. Increase speed of mixer to high and beat to smooth stiff peaks. Stir 1/4 of whites into sauce with rubber spatula. Pour sauce diluted with 1/4 of egg whites inside egg white bowl. Fold in cheese by tablespoonfuls. This should take no longer than 1 minute. Gently scoop mixture into soufflé dish. It should be approximately 3/4 filled. Run finger around rim of dish to set soufflé. Bake in pre-heated 400-degree oven. Immediately reduce oven heat to 375 degrees upon placing soufflé in oven. Bake 35 minutes. Sprinkle 2 tablespoons grated cheese over top and bake 7 to 10 minutes more. Serve immediately.

Nutrient Value per Serving (makes 6 servings): 266.91 calories, 15.35g protein, 7.40g carbohydrates, 19.36g fat

Notes

Fiber-Restricted Diet

Recipes

Sautéed Cocktail Tomatoes
Asparagus with Butter
Steamed Carrots
Bacon-Wrapped Chicken Breasts
Chicken Piccate
Vegetarian Stuffed Peppers
Chicken Breasts with Grapes
Ham Rolls with Eggplant Filling

* * *

The fiber-restricted diet, or low-fiber diet, is the diet of choice for several situations. First, it is an appropriate transitional diet for the person moving from a full liquid to a regular diet. Second, this diet is excellent if the bowel is irritated and the person is experiencing difficulty with cramps, diarrhea, and intestinal pain. The principle of the diet is to slow the movement of the bowel and decrease irritation or inflammation of the tissues. If you are selecting this diet as a lifestyle choice then the advice of your health care provider is essential since extended use of the low-fiber diet could have some nutritional side effects and may contribute to other bowel problems. Nevertheless, it is a great ally in fighting diarrhea and bowel discomfort.

There are some foods you may *NOT* have *AT ALL* on this diet. These are: seeds, nuts, coconut, popcorn, dried beans, peas, lentils, legumes, sauerkraut, winter squash, peas, peanut butter, whole grain(s), flour(s), or other ingredients using whole grains, fruit, or vegetable juice with pulp, bran, dried fruit, all berries, raw fruits, oatmeal, granola, cornbread, graham crackers, and raw eggs.

And there are some foods you may have an unlimited amount of: coffee, tea, milk, sodas and carbonated beverages, fruit drinks, plain sherbet, fruit ices, ice cream, yogurt, custard, gelatin, popsicles, sugar, honey, jelly, plain hard candy, marshmallows, margarine, butter, cream, salad oils, mayonnaise, bacon, plain gravy, salad dressings, meat, fish, chicken, cooked eggs, plain cheeses, boullion, broth and consomme, salt, pepper, spices, herbs, ketchup, mustard.

And of course, there are some foods you may have just some of:

Breads: 1.0 grams of fiber or less per 1 slice or 1-ounce serving. Limit 3 servings per day. These may include refined breads, rolls, biscuits, muffins, crackers, pancakes, waffles, plain pastries, or raisin bread.

Cereals: 1.0 grams of fiber or less per 3/4-cup serving. Limit 1 serving per day. These may include refined cooked cereals (e.g., Cream of Wheat, Cream of Rice, Malt-O-Meal, grits, and Farina) and refined dry cereals (e.g., Cheerios, Cornflakes, Rice Crispies, etc.).

Sweets: 1.0 grams of fiber or less per serving. Limit 1 serving per day.

Fruits: 2.0 grams of fiber or less per 1 cup serving. Limit 1 serving per day. These may include canned or cooked fruits (e.g., apple slices, applesauce, cherries, grapefruit, grapes, oranges, peaches, pineapple, plums) and raw fruits (e.g., bananas, cherries, grapefruit, grapes, melon, oranges, peaches, pineapple).

Fruit juice or vegetable juice containing 0.5 grams of fiber or less per 1-cup serving (no pulp). Limit 2 servings per day.

Potato and potato substitutes: 2.0 grams of fiber or less per 1-cup serving. Limit 1 serving per day. These include cooked white and sweet potatoes without the skin, white rice, and refined pasta.

Soups: 1.0 grams fiber per 6-ounce serving. Limit 1 serving per day. These include bouillon, broth, or cream soups made with allowed foods.

Vegetables: 2.0 grams of fiber or less per 1-cup serving. Limit 2 servings per day. These include the following frozen, canned, cooked or raw vegetables: asparagus, green beans, yellow beans, bean sprouts, beets, cabbage*, carrots, cauliflower*, celery, cucumber*, pared eggplant, collard greens, dandelion greens, mustard greens, green pepper*,

---

*Some people may not do well with these.

lettuce, mushrooms, onion*, rutabaga*, spinach, summer squash, tomato, turnip, zucchini, tomato paste, tomato sauce, and tomato puree.
    Following is a list of foodstuffs included in this diet:

- coffee
- tea
- milk
- sodas and carbonated drinks
- fruit drinks
- plain sherbet
- fruit ices
- ice cream
- yogurt
- custard
- gelatin
- popsicles
- sugar
- honey
- jelly
- plain hard candy
- marshmallows
- margarine
- butter
- cream
- salad oils
- mayonnaise
- bacon
- plain gravy
- salad dressings
- meat
- fish
- chicken
- cooked eggs
- plain cheeses
- bouillon, broth, and consommé
- salt
- pepper
- spices
- herbs
- ketchup
- mustard

SAMPLE RECIPES

Sautéed Cocktail Tomatoes

1 pint cocktail tomatoes
salt and pepper to taste
1 to 2 tablespoons butter
fresh parsley, chopped

Wash tomatoes and pat dry. Melt butter in heavy skillet. Add the tomatoes. Heat through by swirling them around in the skillet. Be careful not to overcook tomatoes or they will burst. Salt and pepper to taste. Remove to a warm bowl. Sprinkle with chopped parsley and serve.

Nutrient Value per Serving (makes 2 servings): 179.98 calories, 3.32g protein, 17.29g carbohydrates, 37.75g fat

Asparagus with Butter

1 pound asparagus
1/3 cup water
1/2 teaspoon salt
2 ounces (1/2 stick) butter, cut into pieces

Wash asparagus and trim stalks as necessary. Slice or leave whole, depending upon preference. Place asparagus in skillet with water and salt. Cover and bring to a strong boil. Boil approximately 1 to 2 minutes. Uncover and add the butter. Return to a strong boil, binding butter and water together. Shake skillet periodically. Boil 20 to 30 seconds. Butter and water will foam. Remove from heat and serve.

Nutrient Value per Serving (makes 2 servings): 285.28 calories, 9.09g protein, 14.44g carbohydrates, 24.09g fat

Steamed Carrots

1 1/2 pounds carrots
2 tablespoons butter
2 tablespoons Madeira wine (optional)
salt and pepper to taste

Wash, peel, and cut carrots into desired shape (e.g., slice, dice, or julienne). Put butter into heavy saucepan and melt. Add carrots. Cover with a tight-fitting lid and place over low heat. Carrots will slowly steam in their own juice. Shake pan periodically to prevent sticking. Cook until tender when pricked with a fork. Carrots are cooked when excess moisture has evaporated. Remove from heat. Salt and pepper to taste. Sprinkle with Madeira if desired.

Nutrient Value per Serving (makes 3 servings): 176.62 calories, 2.59g protein, 23.90g carbohydrates, 8.09g fat

Bacon-Wrapped Chicken Breasts

6 boned, skinned chicken breast halves
1 package dried beef (thinly sliced sandwich beef)
1 16-ounce carton sour cream
1 can cream of mushroom soup
6 slices bacon

Wrap chicken breasts in bacon. Line casserole or baking dish with beef. Place bacon-wrapped chicken breasts on top of beef. Mix sour cream and cream of mushroom soup. Spread sour cream/soup mixture over chicken breasts. Bake uncovered for 3 hours at 275 degrees.

Nutrient Value per Serving (makes 3 servings): 787.11 calories, 70.35g protein, 12.71g carbohydrates, 49.40g fat

Chicken Piccate

4 boned, skinned chicken breast halves
butter and oil
salt and freshly ground pepper
1/4 cup marsala wine
1 tablespoon fresh lemon juice
1/2 cup chicken broth
capers
tarragon

Heat oil and butter in heavy skillet (do not use iron or aluminum). Season chicken with salt and pepper and dredge in flour; shake off excess flour. As soon as butter has stopped foaming, brown chicken on both sides. Do not overcook. Remove chicken to warm platter and cover with foil. Discard excess fat from skillet. Deglaze skillet with the marsala, scraping bottom of skillet (a wire whisk or spoon works well for this). Add chicken broth and lemon juice. Reduce the liquid briefly by cooking. Add the chicken. Add capers and tarragon to taste. Simmer a few minutes over low heat to blend all of the flavors. Serve at once.

Nutrient Value per Serving (makes 2 servings): 579.75 calories, 64.49g protein, 2.17g carbohydrates, 32.56g fat

Vegetarian Stuffed Peppers

2 green (bell) peppers
2 cups prepared white rice (see recipe page 32)
1 6-ounce can tomato paste
1 15-ounce can tomato sauce
cheddar cheese (optional)

Cut green peppers in half. Remove stems and seeds. Rinse. Blanch in boiling water for 3 to 5 minutes. Remove from heat and refresh peppers under cold water. Drain thoroughly. Place blanched pepper halves, open side up, in baking dish. Mix tomato paste with rice. Fill pepper halves with rice mixture. Spoon tomato sauce over stuffed peppers. (Stuffed peppers may be wrapped and frozen at this point. Thaw prior to baking.) Bake at 350 degrees for 30 to 45 minutes. Top with cheddar cheese for the final 10 to 15 minutes of baking if desired.

Nutrient Value per Serving (makes 2 servings): 591.74 calories, 26.69g protein, 82.38g carbohydrates, 20.71g fat

Chicken Breasts with Grapes

1 3/4 pounds boned, skinned chicken breasts
1/2 to 3/4 cup seedless grapes
3 tablespoons butter
salt and pepper to taste
5 teaspoons finely chopped shallots
1/2 cup dry white wine
1 1/2 cups heavy cream

Pound chicken and cut into strips (approximately 1/2-inch wide). Rinse grapes and remove from stem. Heat butter in heavy skillet. Add chicken strips. Cook over high heat, stirring constantly, until chicken is barely cooked (3 to 5 minutes). Remove chicken to warm platter and cover with foil. Add shallots to skillet. Cook briefly until they begin to wilt. Deglaze skillet with white wine, scraping bottom of skillet (a wire whisk or spoon works well for this). Add any juice from chicken platter to wine. Continue cooking until reduced by half. Reduce heat to medium high and add cream, stirring constantly. Add grapes and cook until cream takes on saucelike consistency (4 to 5 minutes). Add salt and pepper. Add chicken and simmer briefly to blend flavors. Try serving this chicken dish with curried rice.

Nutrient Value per Serving (makes 6 servings): 503.41 calories, 42.51g protein, 5.28g carbohydrates, 32.79g fat

Ham Rolls with Eggplant Filling

8 thin slices of baked ham
eggplant filling (see recipe below)
3 tablespoons or more butter
1/4 cup flour
2 1/2 cups milk
salt and pepper to taste
1/8 teaspoon freshly ground nutmeg
cayenne pepper to taste
2 egg yolks
1/4 cup Parmesan or Gruyère cheese, grated

Preheat oven to 425 degrees. Place ham slices on a flat surface. Divide eggplant filling evenly over ham slices in center. Roll up to enclose filling. Butter a baking dish slightly and arrange ham rolls in it. Melt 3 tablespoons butter in saucepan. Add flour, stirring with whisk, to make a light roux. Cook a few minutes to eliminate raw taste. Add milk, stirring constantly. Add salt, pepper, nutmeg, and cayenne pepper. Cook, stirring frequently, about 5 minutes over medium heat. In a small bowl, blend the egg yolks. Add a little of the hot sauce mixture to temper the yolks. Pour tempered yolks into hot sauce mixture and bring to a simmer. Do not let the mixture boil. Pour sauce over ham rolls and top with grated cheese. Place in preheated oven and bake 10 minutes or until hot and bubbling. The top should brown slightly.

Eggplant Filling

1 small eggplant (approximately 1/2 pound)
2 tablespoons butter
1 cup chopped celery
1 cup chopped scallions (green onions), including the green part
1/2 pound cubed whole milk mozzarella cheese

Peel eggplant. Cut into cubes (approximately 2 cups). Melt butter in skillet. When foam has subsided, sauté eggplant, celery, and scallions. Cook about 5 minutes. Remove from heat. Add cheese cubes and blend.

Nutrient Value per Serving (makes 4 servings): 875.16 calories, 77.53g protein, 22.14g carbohydrates, 51.88g fat

Notes

Bananas, Rice, Applesauce, and Tea Diet (B.R.A.T. Diet)

Recipes

White Rice
Applesauce
Curried Rice

* * *

This is not an official diet of any dietetic association as far as we know, but it is a diet heavily employed by those living with HIV or caring for HIV-positive people. This is a very useful diet. The elements are bananas (B), rice (R), applesauce (A), and tea (T). The diet is not meant for long-term use because it is not nutritionally balanced. It is, however, soothing to the mouth and digestive system and aids in calming diarrhea. It is a step up from the clear liquid diet in that it provides some texture and substance to the food and can be combined in truly taste-oriented ways.

SUGGESTIONS

- Try varying the type of tea. Mint, peppermint, and spearmint tea can be very soothing. Also, try a peppermint stick in a cup of regular tea.
- Bananas may be mashed for ease of consumption by individuals with oral pain due to lesions in the mouth or chewing difficulties.
- Applesauce, in large quantities, may actually cause diarrhea, so keep an eye on the amount of pure applesauce consumed.

SAMPLE RECIPES

White Rice

2 cups water
1 cup long grain rice
1 teaspoon salt
1 tablespoon margarine

Bring water, salt, and margarine to a boil in a saucepan. Stir in rice, cover, and reduce heat. Simmer covered until water has been absorbed and rice fluffs (approximately 20 minutes). Fluff rice with a fork prior to serving.

Nutrient Value per Serving (makes 1 serving): 262 calories, 3.5g protein, 35.3g protein, 11.5g fat

Variation: Try serving white rice as a cereal with Vitamite non-dairy, lactose-free beverage mix (prepared according to package directions) and sliced bananas or cinnamon and sugar.

Applesauce

4 medium apples
1/4 cup sugar
1/2 teaspoon cinnamon
1/2 cup water

Pare, core, and slice apples. Combine apples and water in a medium saucepan. Bring to a boil, cover, and simmer 10 minutes or until very tender. Remove from heat. Mash apples until smooth. Add sugar and cinnamon.

Nutrient Value per Serving (makes 2 servings): 259.59 calories, 0.53g protein, 67.21g carbohydrates, 1.0g fat

Curried Rice

1 cup rice
1 small apple, cored
3 tablespoons butter
1/4 to 1/2 cup finely chopped onion
1 clove garlic, minced
2 teaspoons curry powder
1/2 bay leaf
1 1/2 cup chicken broth

Cut apple into quarter-inch cubes (approximately 1 cup). Heat 1 tablespoon butter in saucepan and cook minced garlic and chopped onion until wilted. Add cubed apple and curry powder. Stir. Add rice, bay leaf, and chicken broth. Bring to a boil; cover and cook 17 minutes. Add 1 tablespoon butter and fluff into rice with a fork. Keep rice covered in a warm place until ready to serve.

Nutrient Value per Serving (makes 2 servings): 484 calories, 7.09g protein, 71.19g carbohydrates, 18.45g fat

Notes

Lactose-Free Diet

Recipes

Banana Shake
Cream of Tomato Soup
Frozen Delight
Bean Soup
Black Beans

* * *

Lactose intolerance is a common side condition of HIV and gastrointestinal infections such as rotavirus or giardiasis. The principal symptoms include cramping, diarrhea, stomach pain, and gas occurring fairly rapidly after consuming dairy products. The treatment is avoidance of the offending dairy products and sometimes the use of an enzyme tablet to predigest the lactose in a food. We recommend you discuss with your health care provider your options if you have found lactose intolerance to be an issue for you.

Following is a list of foodstuffs included in this diet:

- Isomil
- Isomil SF
- Mocha Mix
- Nutramigen
- Pregestimil
- Product 3232A RCF
- sodas and other carbonated beverages
- coffees
- teas

- lactose-free formulas such as Ensure, Isocal, Citrotein, Osmo-lyte, Sustacal, Nutri 1000 LF
- fruit juice NOT processed with lactose
- eggs

ABSOLUTELY NO:

- Dairy products including chocolate; condensed, powdered, or dried milk; yogurt; sherbet; Ovaltine (In this case check labels.)

ALLOWABLE IF LACTOSE-FREE:

Breads and Cereals: bread products made without milk, Italian breads, macaroni, spaghetti, soda crackers, rice, and some cooked and cold cereals. Again, in this case, it is best to check the labels of the product you wish to use. Many prepared mixes, biscuits, waffles, pancakes, cereals, and commercial breads and rolls contain lactose or have been prepared with milk solids.

Meat and meat substitutes: kosher hot dogs and cold cuts and meats without lactose. Again, check the package labels. No creamed or breaded meat, fish, or fowl; sausage products; cold cuts containing milk solids; or cheeses are permitted.

Soups: clear, vegetable, consommes, cream soups made with Mocha Mix or nondairy creamers. All the rest are not permitted.

Desserts: water and fruit ices; angel food cake; gelatin; puddings not made with dairy products; cakes, pies, cookies, etc., made from allowed ingredients.

Fats: read labels; this can change from company to company even for the same product. Margarines and salad dressing made without milk(s), oils, shortening, bacon, SOME whipped topping products, butters, nuts, some nondairy creamers. Again the choices are label driven.

Fruits: all fresh, frozen, or canned fruits not processed with lactose.

Vegetables: most fresh, frozen, or canned vegetables are allowed as long as they are not prepared creamed, breaded, or buttered. No instant potatoes, corn curls, or frozen french fries are permitted.

Miscellaneous foods: soy sauce, carob powder, popcorn, olives, pure sugar candy, jelly, marmalade, corn syrup, gravy made with water, baker's cocoa, pickles, pure seasonings and spices, wine, molasses, pure msg, Tofutti frozen dessert, and Sweet 'n' Low are all permissable. Not permitted are chewing gum, some instant coffees, toffee, peppermint, butterscotch, caramels, drug and vitamin preparations if made with lactose, some spice preparations (read labels), and Equal.

SAMPLE RECIPES

Banana Shake

2 ripe bananas
1 can vanilla Ensure (or other lactose-free formula)
ice

Place bananas and Ensure in blender. Fill with ice. Blend until smooth.

Nutrient Value per Serving (makes 1 serving): 459.76 calories, 11.37g protein, 93.35g carbohydrates, 7.09g fat

Variation: Substitute strawberries or other fruit for bananas.

Cream of Tomato Soup

1 14 1/2-ounce can crushed tomatoes
1 1/2 cups prepared Vitamite (or other lactose-free, non-dairy beverage mix)
salt and pepper to taste

Combine ingredients in saucepan and heat thoroughly.

Nutrient Value per Serving (makes 2 servings): 82.22 calories, 3.82g protein, 17.68g carbohydrates, 1.0g fat

Frozen Delight

1 package instant vanilla pudding (lactose-free)
2 cups chilled vanilla Ensure (or other lactose-free formula)
2 cups Cool Whip

Prepare pudding as directed, substituting Ensure for milk. Gently fold in Cool Whip. Pour into freezer container. Cover and freeze until firm.

Nutrient Value per Serving (makes 4 servings): 373.48 calories, 5.65g protein, 34.38g carbohydrates, 16.25g fat

Variation: Substitute chocolate, butterscotch, or other pudding flavors.

Bean Soup

1 20-ounce package Great Northerns (white beans)
1 small onion
2 tablespoons olive oil
1 ham bone with meat
salt and pepper to taste

Soak beans overnight according to package directions. Drain. Place soaked beans and 6 to 8 cups of water in a 5-quart saucepan along with ham bone. Bring to a boil. Cover. Reduce heat and simmer for about 2 hours. Add water as needed to prevent beans from sticking. Chop onion and sauté in olive oil until wilted. Add sautéed onion to beans. Continue cooking beans another hour or until tender. Remove any meat from ham bone and add to beans; discard bone. Salt and pepper to taste.

Nutrient Value per Serving (makes 6 servings): 425.49 calories, 42.21g protein, 21.09g carbohydrates, 18.60g fat

Black Beans

1 pound black beans
1 28-ounce can diced tomatoes
1 10-ounce package frozen spinach
4 carrots
Cajun seasoning

Soak beans overnight according to package instructions. Drain. Place soaked beans in 5-quart saucepan with 6 to 8 cups water. Bring to a boil. Cover and reduce heat. Simmer for about 2 hours, adding more water if needed to prevent beans from sticking. Thaw spinach and drain. Slice carrots. Remove approximately 1 cup beans and mash. Return mashed beans to pot. Add tomatoes, thawed spinach, and sliced carrots. Season with Cajun seasoning to taste. Cover and simmer until beans and carrots are tender, approximately an additional 1 to 2 hours. To serve, mound white rice in middle of bowl and ladle beans over and around rice.

Nutrient Value per Serving (makes 4 servings): 240.18 calories, 14.89g protein, 46.49g carbohydrates, 1.38g fat

Variation: Add cooked chicken cut into bite-sized pieces approximately 30 minutes before serving. Make sure chicken is heated through.

Notes

High-Fiber Diet

Recipes

Marinated Cucumbers
Four-Bean Salad
Baked Onions
Fried Apples
Stewed Tomatoes
Peas with Boston Lettuce
Rice with Leeks
German Potato Salad
24-Hour Fruit Salad
Roasted Potatoes
Spinach and Grapefruit Salad

Sautéed Cocktail Tomatoes and Snow Peas
Peas Paysanne
Cabbage Stew
Shredded Potato Cakes
Brussels Sprouts and Artichokes
Broccoli Casserole
Green Beans with Bacon and Mushrooms
Potato Casserole
Sicilian Potato Casserole
Baked Apples
Red Beans

* * *

Much has been reported in the research literature over the last few years about the benefits of the high-fiber diet as an agent to reduce the risk of cancer(s), and the research looks pretty strong. The increased fiber acts to shorten the time food is in the intestinal tract and to increase the intestinal output. There are many other systemic reactions increasing fiber can cause in the body such as lowering elevated serum carbohydrates, slowing the rate of glucose absorption in the intestine, and lowering blood pressure. For this reason, we urge you to contact your health care provider before switching to this diet for any length of time.

For most, the benefits of the high-fiber diet are great. Increasing the fiber in your diet is a healthy step to progress to, not leap upon, which will help you sustain an overall generally improved state of health. There are, however, some potential side effects to the high-fiber diet. If your fiber load is too high, it may cause cramping, gas, and diarrhea; or, in some rare cases, structural damage to the intestinal tract from the fiber itself. Accordingly, this diet should be approached slowly and steadily; find the right amount of fiber in your diet for you. (For those with inflammation of the bowel, or stenosis of the intestinal lumen, and on some medications, this diet is not approved. Check with your health care provider first.)

Ease into this diet over a period of weeks.

The following foodstuffs are included in this diet:

- whole wheat flour
- bran
- cabbage
- peas
- beans (all kinds)
- apples
- root vegetables
- cereals
- whole grains
- oatmeal and oats
- dried beans
- legumes
- citrus fruits
- strawberries
- wheat
- corn
- graham crackers
- rice
- whole grain pastas
- potatoes
- popcorn
- grits
- asparagus
- broccoli
- carrots
- cauliflower
- greens
- onions
- spinach
- squash
- tomatoes
- lettuce
- peaches
- bananas
- pear
- berries
- nuts

Fats, meats, fish, and eggs may be used for cooking. Most liquids, other than fruit juices, are without fiber unless it is added.

SUGGESTIONS

- Add wheat germ to cereals, yogurt, or ice cream for additional fiber.

• Substitute sweet potatoes for Idaho potatoes. Bake in 400 degree oven 60 to 75 minutes or until done through. Split open and top with butter and cinnamon.

SAMPLE RECIPES

Marinated Cucumbers

2 cucumbers
1 small onion
3/4 cup sugar
3/4 cup vinegar
salt and pepper to taste

Peel and thinly slice cucumbers. Thinly slice onion. Mix all ingredients. Cover and refrigerate several hours. Stir well before serving.

Nutrient Value per Serving (makes 2 servings): 309.17 calories, 0.34g protein, 81.59g carbohydrates, 0.07g fat

Four-Bean Salad

1 can green beans, drained
1 can garbanzo beans, drained
1 can wax beans, drained
1 can kidney beans, drained
1 8-ounce bottle Italian salad dressing

Combine ingredients in large bowl. Cover and refrigerate overnight, stirring occasionally. Serve.

Nutrient Value per Serving (makes 4 servings): 711.46 calories, 25.47g protein, 83.04g carbohydrates, 39.24g fat

Baked Onions

2 to 3 large onions
olive oil
salt

Trim root and point ends off onions. Peel. Slice onion in half horizontally. Brush each half with olive oil and arrange in baking dish. Sprinkle with salt. Bake in 450 degree oven for 30 to 45 minutes or until sweet and tender.

Nutrient Value per Serving (makes 2 servings): 195.34 calories, 2.34g protein, 17.28g carbohydrates, 13.82g fat

Variation: Substitute other vegetables such as mushrooms, zucchini, summer squash, or eggplant. Adjust baking time.

Fried Apples

6 June apples (or other small, tart apples)
1/2 cup sugar
1 tablespoon cinnamon
2 tablespoons bacon grease (or margarine)

Core and quarter apples, leaving peel in tact. Melt bacon grease in skillet. Add apples, sugar, and cinnamon. Sauté over medium-high heat until apples are tender.

Nutrient Value per Serving (makes 4 servings): 276.67 calories, 0.39g protein, 56.65g carbohydrates, 7.15g fat

Stewed Tomatoes

1 29-ounce can sliced tomatoes
1 teaspoon sugar
salt and pepper
1 cup croutons
3 tablespoons margarine

Melt margarine in saucepan over medium heat. Add tomatoes and stir to coat. Add sugar. Stir in croutons. Salt and pepper to taste. Continue to cook until tomatoes are heated through and croutons are soft.

Nutrient Value per Serving (makes 4 servings): 146.89 calories, 3.88g protein, 15.22g carbohydrates, 8.95g fat

Peas with Boston Lettuce

3 tablespoons unsalted butter
12 ounces tiny new or frozen peas
pinch of sugar
1/4 cup water
Boston lettuce cut into chiffonade
salt and pepper to taste

Over medium heat, melt butter in saucepan. Add peas, sugar, and water. Cover and cook till barely tender (2 to 3 minutes). Add lettuce, toss until wilted. Season with salt and pepper to taste.

Nutrient Value per Serving (makes 2 servings): 321.22 calories, 11.71g protein, 30.20g carbohydrates, 18.25g fat

Rice with Leeks

3 leeks
2 cups long grain rice
1 cup water
2 tablespoons margarine
1 teaspoon salt

Trim leeks, leaving ends with some color. Slice trimmed leeks lengthwise just above bulb end. Rinse completely and drain. Cut into half-inch slices. Melt margarine in heavy 2-quart saucepan. Add leeks and sauté until tender. Add salt. Add water and bring to a boil. Add rice, cover, and reduce heat. Simmer 20 minutes or until rice is tender.

Variations: Serve with seafood (e.g., broiled shrimp or baked orange roughy).

Nutrient Value per Serving (makes 2 servings): 537.52 calories, 9.77g protein, 96.83g carbohydrates, 12.36g fat

German Potato Salad

6 medium potatoes
salt and pepper
1 medium onion
1 tablespoon sugar
6 slices bacon
1 tablespoon flour
1/2 cup water
1/2 cup vinegar

Boil potatoes. Peel and slice. Peel onion and chop. Add onion to sliced potatoes. Season with salt and pepper. Fry bacon in heavy skillet. Drain and crumble. Over medium-high heat, add flour to bacon drippings. Cook 2 to 3 minutes, stirring constantly. Add water, vinegar, and sugar. Continue cooking until bubbly. Pour over potatoes. Toss to blend.

Nutrient Value per Serving (makes 4 servings): 328.06 calories, 8.70g protein, 64.33g carbohydrates, 5.06g fat

24-Hour Fruit Salad

2 cups Royal Anne cherries (halved, drained)
2 cups pineapple chunks (drained)
2 large oranges (remove sections and cut in pieces)
2 cups marshmallows
1 cup whipped cream
Place ingredients in a large bowl.

Dressing:

In top of a double boiler, put 2 whole eggs. Beat well. Add 4 tablespoons of vinegar, 4 tablespoons sugar, and continue beating while cooking until thick. Remove from heat and add 4 tablespoons butter. Stir until butter is melted. Cool. Fold whipped cream into dressing and add to drained fruit and marshmallows. Place in a bowl and let stand for 24 hours or longer covered in the refrigerator.

Nutrient Value per Serving (makes 4 servings): 361.32 calories, 3.22g protein, 48.15g carbohydrates, 19.54g fat

Roasted Potatoes

4 Idaho potatoes
1/2 teaspoon salt
1/2 teaspoon freshly ground pepper
4 tablespoons unsalted butter
1 tablespoon vegetable oil
water

Peel potatoes (optional) and cut each into slices about 1 inch thick. Place slices, with flat sides down, in one large or two small iron skillets. Do not overlap slices. Sprinkle with salt and pepper. Add butter, bit by bit, placed around slices. Add oil. Add just enough water to almost cover potato slices. Bring to a rolling boil on top of stove and then place into a pre-heated 425-degree oven. Bake for 35 to 40 minutes. Water should evaporate and potatoes will sizzle in oil and butter mixture. Remove from oven and check to see if slices are browned on bottom. If not, place skillet on direct heat on top of stove for a few minutes. Brush with additional butter when serving if desired.

Nutrient Value per Serving (makes 4 servings): 248.03 calories, 2.44g protein, 27.01g carbohydrates, 15.06g fat

Spinach and Grapefruit Salad

Wash and stem fresh spinach. Cut grapefruit into chunks. Set aside. When ready to serve, toss with poppy seed dressing (see recipe below).

Note: For 4 people, allow approximately 2 pounds fresh spinach and 1 large grapefruit.

Poppy Seed Dressing

3 tablespoons white wine or champagne vinegar
3 tablespoons honey
juice of 1 lemon
1/4 cup olive oil
1/2 cup vegetable oil
1/4 cup poppy seeds
1 teaspoon pepper
approximately 1/2 teaspoon salt

Toast poppy seeds in skillet. Blend with remaining ingredients (whisk together or shake in sealed container).

Nutrient Value per Serving (makes 4 servings): 540.26 calories, 9.40g protein, 27.03g carbohydrates, 46.75g fat

Variation: Substitute fresh strawberries for grapefruit.

Sautéed Cocktail Tomatoes and Snow Peas

2 tablespoons butter
1 pint cocktail tomatoes
2 scallions, sliced
1 tablespoon chopped parsley
1/2 pound snow peas
1/2 teaspoon dried basil

Trim snow peas and cut diagonally. Melt butter in large skillet over high heat. Add cut snow peas and toss in butter for 1 minute. Add all other ingredients and sauté quickly until heated through. Serve at once.

Nutrient Value per Serving (makes 2 servings): 206.12 calories, 6.06g protein, 20.87g carbohydrates, 12.38g fat

Peas Paysanne

1 shallot, minced
14 to 16 ounces frozen peas
1 cup shredded lettuce
5 slices bacon
3 to 4 tablespoons butter
1 teaspoon sugar
1/2 teaspoon salt
1 tablespoon cornstarch
2 tablespoons water

Thaw frozen peas. Fry bacon, crumble, and set aside. Place a large heavy sauté pan over medium heat. Melt butter, sauté shallot until soft. Sprinkle sugar over shallot and let the mixture brown slightly. Add the peas and salt. Stir mixture. Push the peas around the rim of the pan, forming a circle. Leave center empty. Cover, turn heat to low and cook 5 minutes. Add the shredded lettuce, placing it in the center. Cover and let wilt for about 2 minutes. Add the bacon bits, stir together. Cover and cook a few minutes more. Pour juices from pan into small bowl. Dissolve cornstarch in 2 tablespoons water and pour into juices. Pour cornstarch mixture over peas. Stir. Remove from heat, cover, and let stand a few more minutes. Serve.

Nutrient Value per Serving (makes 2 servings): 340.14 calories, 9.69g protein, 19.47g carbohydrates, 25.35g fat

Cabbage Stew

1 head cabbage
2 cups stewed tomatoes
2 cups water
1 pound ground beef
1 package onion soup mix
1 tablespoon brown sugar
1 tablespoon sugar
salt and pepper to taste

Brown ground beef. Core and slice cabbage. Combine all ingredients and simmer until cabbage is tender.

Nutrient Value per Serving (makes 2 servings): 868.81 calories, 70.05g protein, 51.94g carbohydrates, 41.32g fat

Variations: Add peeled potatoes or rice during cooking. Add sausage in addition to, or in place of, ground beef.

Shredded Potato Cakes

4 large baking potatoes
1/2 onion
2 eggs
2 tablespoons flour
2 tablespoons milk
salt and pepper to taste
2 tablespoons melted butter
clarified butter for sauté

Grate the potatoes (this may be done using a food processor with a large grating blade). Grate the onion and mix with the potatoes. Place in a bowl. Blend the eggs, flour, milk, melted butter, salt, and pepper thoroughly. Pour over potatoes and toss. Heat clarified butter in large, heavy skillet. Measure out approximately 1/4 cup of the potatoes and place in skillet. Flatten into cake and sauté until golden brown. Serve at once.

Nutrient Value per Serving (makes 4 servings): 388.66 calories, 8.87g protein, 57.16g carbohydrates, 14.45g fat

Brussels Sprouts and Artichokes

1 10-ounce package frozen Brussels sprouts
1/2 cup water
1 14-ounce can artichoke hearts, drained
2/3 cup mayonnaise
1/2 teaspoon celery salt
1/4 cup Parmesan cheese
1/4 cup margarine, melted
2 teaspoons lemon juice
1/4 cup sliced almonds

Cook Brussels sprouts in 1/2 cup water until tender. Drain. Cut Brussels sprouts in half; cut artichoke hearts in quarters. Put into greased 1-quart casserole. Combine remaining ingredients and spoon over vegetables. Bake uncovered at 425 degrees for 10 to 15 minutes.

Nutrient Value per Serving (makes 4 servings): 568.51 calories, 9.80g protein, 16.84g carbohydrates, 54.64g fat

Broccoli Casserole

1 package frozen chopped broccoli
1/2 cup celery soup
1/2 cup grated sharp cheddar cheese
1 egg, well beaten
1/2 cup mayonnaise (do not substitute salad dressing)
1 tablespoon grated onion
salt and pepper to taste
1/2 cup cheese or Ritz cracker crumbs

Cook broccoli 5 minutes. Drain. Combine other ingredients, except cracker crumbs, to make sauce. Combine sauce with broccoli. Pour into casserole. Sprinkle the top with cracker crumbs. Bake at 400 degrees for approximately 30 minutes. May be refrigerated or frozen before baking.

Nutrient Value per Serving (makes 4 servings): 576.64 calories, 21.59g protein, 14.31g carbohydrates, 49.55g fat

Green Beans with Bacon and Mushrooms

12 slices bacon
1 cup chopped onion
2 (4 1/2-ounce) cans sliced mushrooms, drained
3 (9-ounce) packages frozen sliced green beans
1 tablespoon sugar
salt and pepper to taste

Cook bacon in large skillet. Remove and crumble. Reserve 1 table-spoon bacon grease in pan. Sauté onion in bacon grease. Add mushrooms and sauté another 2 minutes. Add green beans, sugar, and 2 tablespoons water. Cover and cook 10 minutes or more. Add crumbled bacon and salt and pepper to taste. Mix gently and serve.

Nutrient Value per Serving (makes 3 servings): 236.1 calories, 11.92g protein, 20.65g carbohydrates, 12.97g fat

Potato Casserole

Casserole

1 32-ounce package hash browns thawed
1 1/2 to 2 cups shredded cheese
1 cup sour cream
1 stick margarine, melted
1 can cream of chicken soup
1 can cream of potato soup
salt and pepper to taste

Topping

2 cups crushed cornflakes
1/2 stick margarine, melted

Mix all ingredients for casserole in 9 x 13-inch pan. Mix topping ingredients and spread evenly over casserole. Bake at 350 degrees for 75 minutes.

Nutrient Value per Serving (makes 6 servings): 850.65 calories, 17.95g protein, 55.99g carbohydrates, 63.96g fat

Sicilian Potato Casserole

3/4 cup sliced pepperoni
4 baking potatoes, peeled and thinly sliced
1 teaspoon minced garlic
1/2 red bell pepper, chopped
1/2 green bell pepper, chopped
1/4 cup black olives, chopped
1/2 cup grated Parmesan cheese
salt and pepper to taste
1 cup heavy cream

Line bottom of one-quart casserole with sliced pepperoni. Add a layer of sliced potatoes, garlic, red and green peppers, black olives, Parmesan cheese, and salt and pepper to taste. Top with another layer and continue adding layers until all ingredients are used. Pour in the heavy cream. Seal tightly with aluminum foil and bake at 350 degrees for 45 to 60 minutes until bubbly and golden brown.

Nutrient Value per Serving (makes 4 servings): 587.35 calories, 14.72g protein, 55.54g carbohydrates, 34.97g fat

Baked Apples

4 to 6 large baking apples
1 1/2 to 2 cups raisins
1 cup sugar
1 cup water
1/2 teaspoon ground nutmeg
1/2 teaspoon cinnamon
2 tablespoons butter

Core apples and pare a strip from the top of each. Place in a baking dish. Fill apples with raisins. Combine sugar, water, nutmeg, and cinnamon. Pour over apples. Dot with butter. Bake uncovered in 350-degree oven for approximately 1 hour. Baste apples with pan juices occasionally throughout baking.

Nutrient Value per Serving (makes 4 servings): 649.53 calories, 3.01g protein, 155.96g carbohydrates, 7.24g fat

Red Beans

1 pound dried red kidney beans
1 medium onion
1 medium green pepper
2 to 3 cloves garlic
3 to 4 tablespoons olive oil
1 28-ounce can diced tomatoes
1 pound smoked pork sausage such as Polish sausage, kielbasa, or andouille
Cajun seasoning to taste

Soak beans overnight according to package directions. Drain. Place soaked beans and 6 to 8 cups water in 5-quart saucepan. Bring to a boil. Cover. Reduce heat and simmer for about 2 hours, adding more water as necessary to prevent beans from sticking. Chop onion, green pepper, and garlic; sauté in olive oil. Remove approximately 1 cup beans and mash. Return mashed beans to pot. Add sautéed onion, green pepper, and garlic. Add tomatoes. Season with Cajun seasoning to taste. Cover and simmer an additional hour. Cut sausage into bite-sized pieces, brown in skillet, and add to beans. Cover and simmer until beans are tender and sausage is heated through. To serve, mound white rice in middle of bowl and ladle beans over and around rice.

Nutrient Value per Serving (makes 6 servings): 422.30 calories, 16.07g protein, 20.01g carbohydrates, 31.30g fat

Notes

Bland Diet

Recipes

Raspberry Float
Pasta Salad
Easy Tortellini Soup
Creamy Chicken Noodle Soup
Broccoli and Cheese Soup
One-Eyed Egyptians
Creamy Potato Soup

Noodle Pudding
Baked Egg Noodles
Dumplings
Watercress Soup
Sour Cream Coffee Cake
German Potato Dumplings

* * *

By the name alone this diet sounds like a big bore and hardly one that could entice a person to eat. But, such is not really the case. (Just look at the recipes!). This diet is really not a list of foods to eat; it is a list of a few items to avoid, then you can go to town with the foods you may have. Here are the foods to avoid: caffeine (C), alcohol (A), pepper (P), spice (S)—(aka CAPS free). Basically anything that would be irritating to the intestinal tract and stomach is off limits. Some folks recommend eliminating citrus fruits, tomato and tomato juice, and heavy amounts of fats and peppermint as well. If you are on a bland diet or would like to try it, we recommend strictly adhering to the diet at first then gradually (and that does mean slowly over days, not meals) add in one item at a time to find what foods can be tolerated and what cannot. You may want to begin this diet with hot cereals such as Cream of Wheat or oatmeal and gradually progress to other foods from there.

SUGGESTIONS

- Try hot cereals that are generally soothing to the stomach and intestine such as Cream of Wheat, oatmeal, or Wheatena. Prepare according to package directions.
- Try plain pasta cooked according to package instructions and tossed lightly with a small amount of butter or margarine.
- Try couscous as an alternative to traditional pasta or rice.

SAMPLE RECIPES

Raspberry Float

3 scoops raspberry sherbet
3/4 to 1 cup ginger ale

Place sherbet and ginger ale in blender or drink mixer. Blend until smooth. (Adjust amount of ginger ale for desired thickness.)

Nutrient Value per Serving (makes 2 servings): 308.81 calories, 4.66g protein, 42.0g carbohydrates, 14.63g fat

Variation: Substitute other sherbet flavors such as orange, pineapple, or lime.

Pasta Salad

1 16-ounce package pasta shells
1 16-ounce carton sour cream
1 10-ounce package frozen mixed vegetables
salt to taste

Cook pasta according to package directions. Drain. Thaw vegetables and drain. Mix cooked pasta, sour cream, and vegetables. Salt to taste. Refrigerate and serve.

Nutrient Value per Serving (makes 4 servings): 467.19 calories, 12.90g protein, 49.38g carbohydrates, 25.13g fat

Easy Tortellini Soup

1 9-ounce package fresh tortellini
4 cups fresh or canned chicken broth

Bring chicken broth to a boil in large saucepan. Cook tortellini in chicken broth for 7 to 8 minutes or until tender. Ladle into bowls. Top with fresh Parmesan cheese if desired.

Nutrient Value per Serving (makes 4 servings): 226.71 calories, 10.79g protein, 30.58g carbohydrates, 5.82g fat

Creamy Chicken Noodle Soup

4 cups fresh or canned chicken broth
1 cup milk
1 cup cooked, chopped chicken (fresh or canned)
1 cup enriched egg noodles

Bring chicken broth to a boil in a large saucepan. Add noodles and cook until tender. Reduce heat. Add chicken and milk. Cook until chicken is heated through.

Nutrient Value per Serving (makes 4 servings): 186.28 calories, 17.57g protein, 14.29g carbohydrates, 6.02g fat

Broccoli and Cheese Soup

2 tablespoons finely chopped onion
2 tablespoons margarine or butter
3 tablespoons flour
1/2 teaspoon salt
1/8 teaspoon pepper
2 cups milk
1 cup shredded American cheese
2 chicken bouillon cubes
1 bay leaf
1 1/2 cups water
1 10-ounce package frozen chopped broccoli

Cook onion in butter or margarine in large saucepan until tender. Stir in flour, salt, and pepper until well blended. Add milk all at once. Cook until thickened, stirring constantly, about 1 minute. Add cheese and stir until melted. Remove from heat. In a medium saucepan, dissolve bouillon cubes in water. Add bay leaf. Bring to a boil. Add broccoli and cook according to package directions; do not drain. Add broccoli and cooking liquid to cheese mixture. Stir until well blended. Remove bay leaf and serve.

Nutrient Value per Serving (makes 4 servings): 313.97 calories, 16.42g protein, 14.80g carbohydrates, 21.80g fat

One-Eyed Egyptians

bread slices
margarine
eggs

Melt margarine in heavy skillet. Cut round hole in center of bread slices with biscuit cutter. Place bread slices in hot skillet. Drop an egg into each hole. Cook as for fried egg, turning to cook both sides. Add additional margarine if needed. Fry bread rounds and serve on the side.

Nutrient Value per Serving (per slice): 241.31 calories, 8.55g protein, 13g carbohydrates, 17.49g fat

Creamy Potato Soup

10 slices bacon
4 tablespoons margarine
1 cup finely chopped onion
6 cups potatoes (peeled and cubed)
2 cans cream of chicken soup
4 cups milk
salt and pepper

Fry bacon until crisp. Drain. Place margarine in heavy saucepan. Add onions and sauté over medium-high heat until wilted. Add potatoes and enough water to cover (1 to 2 cups). Cover and cook until potatoes are tender (approximately 20 minutes). Combine chicken soup and milk. Add to potato mixture. Heat through, but do not boil. Salt and pepper to taste. Crumble bacon into soup and serve.

Nutrient Value per Serving (makes 4 servings): 590.1 calories, 19.26g protein, 51.37g carbohydrates, 34.83g fat

Noodle Pudding

1/4 cup margarine
8 ounces egg noodles
2 eggs
1/2 cup sugar
1/8 teaspoon cinnamon
pinch of salt
grated rind of half a lemon
1/2 cup raisins

Preheat oven to 375 degrees. Place margarine in a 10 x 8- or 8-inch round baking dish and place in oven. Cook noodles according to package directions. Drain well. Whisk eggs and sugar together. Add cinnamon, salt, grated lemon rind, and raisins to egg mixture. Stir to blend. Stir in the noodles and melted margarine (be sure to swirl margarine in dish to coat sides). Pour noodle mixture into baking dish. Bake in 375-degree oven for 45 minutes or until set in the middle and brown on top.

Nutrient Value per Serving (makes 4 servings): 409 calories, 12g protein, 55g carbohydrates, 16g fat

Baked Egg Noodles

8 ounces egg noodles
3 tablespoons margarine
1/2 cup partially crushed croutons

Cook noodles according to package directions. Drain well. Rub 10 x 8- or 8-inch round baking dish with 1 tablespoon margarine. Pour noodles into greased baking dish. Dot noodles with remaining 2 tablespoons margarine. Top with partially crushed croutons. Bake in 350-degree oven for 15 minutes or until heated through.

Nutrient Value per Serving (makes 4 servings): 322 calories, 9g protein, 45g carbohydrates, 12g fat

Dumplings

2 cans chicken broth
1 7 1/2-ounce can regular biscuits
1/2 cup flour
salt and pepper to taste

Bring chicken broth to a boil in a large saucepan. Cut raw biscuits into quarters. Dredge in flour. Add biscuits and any remaining flour to boiling chicken broth. Add salt and pepper. Reduce heat and simmer for 10 minutes uncovered, stirring occassionally. Cover and simmer an additional 10 minutes. Stir and serve.

Nutrient Value per Serving (makes 4 servings): 226 calories, 8g protein, 36g carbohydrates, 9g fat

Variation: Substitute beef broth.

Watercress Soup

3 leeks, diced
1 1/2 pounds zucchini, peeled and diced
1 tablespoon butter
4 cups chicken broth
1 bunch watercress (may substitute a handful of fresh spinach)
1/3 cup heavy cream

Heat butter in a 4-quart pan. Add diced leeks and cook until soft. Add zucchini and sauté for about 3 minutes. Do not brown. Add chicken broth and simmer until zucchini is tender. Season to taste with salt. Bring soup to a boil and add watercress. Simmer for 2 minutes. Pour into blender or food processor and blend until smooth. Add the cream just before serving.

Nutrient Value per Serving (makes 4 servings): 192.11 calories, 4.21g protein, 19.84g carbohydrates, 11.66g fat

Sour Cream Coffee Cake

2 cups sugar
2 sticks margarine
2 cups flour
1/2 teaspoon salt
1 teaspoon baking powder
2 eggs
8 ounces sour cream
1/2 teaspoon vanilla
1/2 cup brown sugar
1 teaspoon cinnamon
1/2 cup chopped nuts
1 cup powdered sugar
3 tablespoons milk

Grease and flour a tube pan. Preheat oven to 350 degrees. Cream sugar and butter in large bowl. Add eggs one at a time, beating after each. Sift dry ingredients together. Add dry ingredients alternately with sour cream to creamed mixture. Add vanilla. Pour half of batter into tube pan. Mix brown sugar, cinnamon, and nuts; sprinkle over batter. Pour remaining batter over nut mixture. Bake approximately 50 minutes or until done. Invert tube pan and remove cake from pan. Mix milk with powdered sugar. Drizzle glaze over cake while cake is still warm.

Nutrient Value per Serving (makes 8 servings): 936.64 calories, 6.89g protein, 102.97g carbohydrates, 57.20g fat

German Potato Dumplings

2 cups prepared mashed potatoes
1 cup fresh bread crumbs
1 teaspoon salt
1 egg
1 cup flour
1/2 cup butter, melted
pepper

Combine mashed potatoes, bread crumbs, salt, pepper, and egg. Mix well. Knead on a floured board until firm. Knead in more flour as necessary. Dough must not stick to hands. When dough is firm, form into a ball and place on a saucer. Pinch off small finger-size pieces and drop into an open kettle of boiling salted water. Boil 5 minutes or until dumplings puff and rise to top of water. Remove from water and drain. Arrange dumplings on a platter. Pour melted butter over dumplings.

Nutrient Value per Serving (makes 2 servings): 1,031.23 calories, 20.39g protein, 121.25g carbohydrates, 53.12g fat

Notes

High-Protein/High-Calorie Diet

Recipes

Garlic Pasta
Beef and Rice Creole
Macaroni and Cheese Casserole
Sauerkraut and Noodles
Beef Noodle Casserole
Beef Stew
Hot Brown
Egg Casserole
Hot Crossed Tuna Casserole
Baked Stuffed Tomatoes
French Onion Soup
Egg Cassoulets
Spinach Cheese Pie
Broccoli Mushroom Quiche
24-Hour Wine and Cheese Omelet
Russian-Style Breast of Chicken
Shredded Potato Cakes
Tournedos of Beef with Shallot Sauce

Garnished Sauerkraut
Bread Pudding with Whiskey Sauce
Apple Cake
Prune Cake
Banana Nut Bread
Traditional White Bread
Apple Coffee Cake
Ice Box Rolls
Butterscotch Pie
Chocolate Fudge
Peanut Butter Fudge
Cherry Cobbler
Rice Pudding
Chocolate Pie
Strawberry Pie
Pineapple Coconut Cake
Banana Pudding
Coconut Pie

* * *

This is not just an eat-all-you-want diet, even though, as you look at the calories, it may seem that way. The diet is actually made to provide a minimum of 1.5 grams of protein per kilogram of body weight daily. The primary purposes of this diet are to work to prevent wasting, to build up energy resources while decreasing energy loss, and to replenish the physical resources. The benefits of this diet are truly health-oriented for the HIV-positive individual. The increased calories and nutritional content assist in improving and maintaining the immune system; stopping and possibly reversing tissue wasting and weight loss; and assisting in wound healing. We know severe weight loss is strongly associated with mortality in HIV; this diet is a positive step in fighting weight loss and tissue wasting syndromes. It is important to note that the high protein and high calories must go together to achieve the results you want. And, as always, if you plan to be on this diet for a long period of time, it is important that you consult your health care provider first. (Note: This diet should not be used if you are experiencing liver disease, kidney disease, or have a calcium balance problem.)

Approach this diet slowly and work up to total protein and calorie intake.

Suggestion

- Add chopped hard-boiled eggs to to dishes for additional protein.

SAMPLE RECIPES

Garlic Pasta

4 to 5 cloves garlic
1 9-ounce package angel-hair pasta
1 tablespoon olive oil
3 to 4 tablespoons butter
1/4 to 1/2 cup grated Parmesan cheese
3 to 4 tablespoons crushed red pepper

Skin and chop garlic. Fill large saucepan with water. Bring water to a boil over high heat. Add garlic, olive oil, and pasta. Cook pasta according to package directions or until al dente. Drain thoroughly. Toss with butter, Parmesan cheese, and crushed red pepper.

Nutrient Value per Serving (makes 4 servings): 393.34 calories, 14.17g protein, 40.03g carbohydrates, 20.72g fat

Beef and Rice Creole

1/4 cup chopped green pepper
1/4 cup chopped onion
1 pound ground beef
1 1-pound canned stewed tomatoes
1/2 cup hot water
2/3 cup white rice
salt and pepper

Place ground beef, chopped green pepper, and chopped onion in heavy saucepan. Over medium heat, brown ground beef and sauté green pepper and onion. Reduce temperature and simmer approximately 5 minutes. Add tomatoes, hot water, and rice. Cover and cook 15 to 20 minutes or until rice is tender and flavors are blended. Salt and pepper to taste.

Nutrient Value per Serving (makes 2 servings): 829.8 calories, 70.3g protein, 42.96g carbohydrates, 40.84g fat

Macaroni and Cheese Casserole

1 16-ounce package shredded sharp cheddar cheese
1 8-ounce box elbow macaroni
4 tablespoons margarine
1/2 cup cracker crumbs
1/4 cup milk
salt and pepper to taste

Cook macaroni according to package instructions. Drain. Layer half of macaroni in an 8 x 8-inch Pyrex baking dish. Sprinkle with salt and pepper. Top with half of the cheese. Dot with half of the margarine. Repeat for second layer. Sprinkle cracker crumbs on top and add milk. Bake in 475-degree oven for approximately 15 minutes or until cheese melts and top browns.

Nutrient Value per Serving (makes 4 servings): 795 calories, 37g protein, 52g carbohydrates, 52g fat

Sauerkraut and Noodles

1 pound bacon
1 29-ounce can sauerkraut
2 medium onions
1 8-ounce package Pennsylvania Dutch noodles
salt and pepper to taste
sugar

Cut bacon into pieces and saute. Pour off most of the fat. Slice onions and add to bacon. Continue to sauté until onions wilt. Add sauerkraut and 1/2 can of water. Simmer while cooking noodles. Salt and pepper to taste; add a sprinkle of sugar. Cook noodles according to package instructions. Drain noodles. Mix with sauerkraut. Put in 9 x 13-inch casserole and bake in 350-degree oven for 1 to 1 1/2 hours.

Nutrient Value per Serving (makes 4 servings): 777.95 calories, 39.13g protein, 25.93g carbohydrates, 4.65g fat

Beef Noodle Casserole

2 cans stewed tomatoes
1 package onion soup mix
10 ounces egg noodles
1 1/2 pounds ground beef

Cook egg noodles according to package directions. Drain. Brown ground beef. Remove excess grease. Add all ingredients to browned ground beef. Top with grated cheddar cheese. Bake at 375 degrees for 45 minutes.

Nutrient Value per Serving (makes 4 servings): 680.02 calories, 54.43g protein, 41.02g carbohydrates, 31.50g fat

Beef Stew

3 1/2 pounds beef (cubed)
3 to 4 tablespoons cooking oil
2 cloves garlic
1 pound carrots
4 small onions
1 10-ounce package frozen peas
2 to 3 medium potatoes
4 beef bouillon cubes
4 cups water
1 bay leaf
salt and pepper

Peel and chop garlic. Place cooking oil in a heavy saucepan. Add beef and brown over high heat. When beef is almost brown, add garlic. Be careful not to burn garlic. Add water, bouillon, and bay leaf. Cover. Reduce heat and simmer 60 to 75 minutes or until beef is tender. Peel and slice carrots. Peel and slice onions. Peel potatoes and cut into bite-sized cubes. Add carrots, onions, and potatoes to stew. Adjust water if necessary, but be careful not to dilute stew. Continue simmering for 45 to 50 minutes or until vegetables are almost done. Add frozen peas and cook 5 minutes more. Remove bay leaf. Salt and pepper to taste.

Nutrient Value per Serving (makes 4 servings): 1,189.0 calories, 132.92g protein, 40.81g carbohydrates, 51.99g fat

Hot Brown

4 slices of toasted whole grain or enriched bread
8 slices of turkey
8 slices of ham
8 slices of bacon
2 tablespoons margarine
2 tablespoons flour
1/4 teaspoon salt
1 cup milk
1/2 cup shredded cheddar cheese
Parmesan cheese

Fry bacon until crisp. Drain. Arrange toast slices in oven-proof dish. Place ham and turkey on toast slices. Melt margarine in saucepan over medium-high heat. Add flour. Cook briefly, stirring constantly. Add salt and milk. Continue to cook, stirring constantly, until sauce begins to thicken. Add cheese and cook, stirring constantly, until melted. Ladle cheese sauce over top of turkey. Sprinkle lightly with Parmesan cheese. Bake in 450-degree oven until brown. Remove from oven. Place 2 strips of crisp bacon on top of each hot brown.

Nutrient Value per Serving (makes 4 servings): 452.88 calories, 35.13g protein, 19.60g carbohydrates, 25.61g fat

Egg Casserole

1/2 cup chopped onion
2 tablespoons margarine
2 tablespoons flour
1 1/4 cups milk
1 cup sharp cheddar shredded cheese
6 hard-boiled eggs, sliced or quartered
1 1/2 cups crushed potato chips
10-12 slices bacon

Fry bacon until crisp. Drain and crumble. Cook onion in margarine until tender but not brown. Blend in flour, add milk, and cook, stirring constantly, until mixture thickens. Add cheese and continue cooking, stirring constantly, until cheese is melted. Remove from heat. Place layer of egg slices in 10 x 6-inch baking dish. Cover with half of cheese sauce, half of potato chips, and half of bacon. Repeat layer. Bake in 350-degree oven for 30 minutes.

Nutrient Value per Serving (makes 4 servings): 821.88 calories, 30.25g protein, 45.53g carbohydrates, 58.32g fat

Hot Crossed Tuna Casserole

2 6 1/2- or 7-ounce cans of tuna, drained
1 10-ounce package frozen peas, thawed
1 cup shredded cheddar cheese
1 cup celery slices
1/2 cup bread crumbs
1/4 cup chopped onion
1/4 teaspoon salt
1/8 teaspoon pepper
1 cup Miracle Whip salad dressing
1 8-ounce can crescent dinner rolls

Combine tuna, peas, cheese, celery, bread crumbs, onion, seasonings, and 1 cup salad dressing. Mix well. Spoon into a 10 x 6-inch baking dish. Separate dough into 2 rectangles; press perforations to seal. Cut dough into 4 long and 8 short strips. Place strips over casserole in lattice design. Brush lightly with salad dressing and sprinkle with sesame seeds. Bake in 350-degree oven for 35 to 40 minutes or until golden brown.

Nutrient Value per Serving (makes 4 servings): 874.31 calories, 47.21g protein, 86.24g carbohydrates, 36.42g fat

Baked Stuffed Tomatoes

6 tomatoes
1/2 cup whole grain or enriched bread crumbs
1 to 2 garlic cloves, mashed
1 tablespoon parsley
2 tablespoons margarine, melted
3 tablespoons onion
1 tablespoon oregano
1/8 teaspoon thyme
1/4 teaspoon salt and pepper
olive oil

Trim tops from tomatoes. Leave skin in tact. Seed tomatoes. Blend bread crumbs, mashed garlic, parsley, margarine, onion, oregano, thyme, salt, and pepper. Stuff tomatoes and place in greased baking dish. Bake in 400-degree oven for 10 minutes.

Nutrient Value per Serving (makes 4 servings): 198.12 calories, 3.7g protein, 17.71g carbohydrates, 13.67g fat

French Onion Soup

8 to 10 medium-size onions
1/2 cup margarine
3 cans beef bouillon
1/2 cup dry sherry or red wine
salt and pepper
1 loaf French bread
Gruyère, Swiss, or Parmesan cheese

Peel onions. Slice whole onions to form rings, discarding ends. Place sliced onions and margarine in large stock pot. Cover and sauté over medium-low heat until tender but not brown. Add beef bouillon and 3 cans water. Add sherry or red wine. Cover and simmer over low heat for 2 to 3 hours (the longer the better). Salt and pepper to taste. Tear approximately 1/4 loaf of French bread into chunks and stir into soup. Place a French bread chunk with crust in the bottom of each individual oven-proof bowl or ramekin that is to be used for soup. Ladle soup over bread crust. Top with Gruyère cheese (fresh Parmesan or Swiss may be substituted). Place under broiler until cheese is bubbly and begins to brown. Serve with remaining French bread.

Nutrient Value per Serving (makes 6 servings): 825.92 calories, 24.05g protein, 46.27g carbohydrates, 22.11g fat

Egg Cassoulets

2 English muffins (4 halves)
6 eggs
8 slices bacon
2 tablespoons margarine
2 tablespoons flour
1/4 teaspoon salt
1/8 to 1/4 teaspoon fresh grated nutmeg
1 cup milk
1/2 cup shredded Swiss cheese

Toast English muffins. Fry bacon until crisp; drain well; crumble. Hard boil eggs; peel; cut in half lengthwise. Place toasted English muffin halves in bottoms of 4 individual cassolettes. Arrange 3 hard-boiled egg halves on top of each English muffin half. Melt margarine in saucepan over medium-high heat. Add flour. Cook briefly, stirring constantly. Add salt and milk. Continue to cook, stirring constantly, until sauce begins to thicken. Add cheese and cook, stirring constantly, until melted. Add nutmeg. Ladle cheese sauce over eggs. Top with crumbled bacon. Bake in 450-degree oven 15 to 20 minutes or until sauce is bubbly and eggs are heated through.

Nutrient Value per Serving (makes 4 servings): 479.80 calories, 28.0g protein, 21.29g carbohydrates, 30.84g fat

Spinach Cheese Pie

1/3 cup chopped onion
2 tablespoons margarine
1 pound sliced Swiss cheese
1/2 pound sliced cheddar cheese
1 10-ounce package frozen chopped spinach
3 eggs
1 3/4 cup milk
3 tablespoons flour
salt and pepper to taste
1 9-inch pie shell

Thaw spinach and drain well. Cook onion in margarine until soft and wilted; cool. Arrange Swiss cheese in pie shell. Top with cheddar followed with drained spinach and then sautéed onions. Beat eggs, flour, salt, and pepper together. Add milk and whisk to blend. Pour over ingredients in pie shell. Bake in 325-degree oven for 60 to 75 minutes or until knife inserted in center comes out clean.

Nutrient Value per Serving (makes 6 servings): 731.69 calories, 40.34g protein, 27.35g carbohydrates, 51.46g fat

Broccoli Mushroom Quiche

1 9-inch pie crust, unbaked
1 10-ounce package frozen broccoli spears
6 mushrooms
1 1/2 pounds Swiss cheese
3 eggs
3 tablespoons flour
1 3/4 cups milk
salt and pepper to taste
4 slices bacon

Line quiche pan or pie pan with pie crust. Prick bottom with fork and bake according to directions until lightly browned. Cool. Fry bacon and drain. Thaw broccoli and drain. Clean mushrooms and slice in half. Slice Swiss cheese. Line pie crust with single layer of cheese. Arrange broccoli and mushrooms on top of single layer of cheese. Top with remaining Swiss cheese. In a deep bowl, whisk eggs until blended. Add flour, salt, and pepper. Whisk to blend. Add milk and whisk to blend. Pour egg and milk mixture over cheese. Top with crumbled bacon. Bake quiche in 325-degree oven for 60 to 75 minutes or until knife inserted in middle comes out clean.

Nutrient Value per Serving (makes 6 servings): 709.89 calories, 42.80g protein, 27.52g carbohydrates, 47.73g fat

Variation: Substitute other vegetables; add meats, poultry, or sea-food.

24-Hour Wine and Cheese Omelet

1 large loaf day-old French or Italian bread
6 tablespoons unsalted butter, melted
3/4 pound Swiss cheese, shredded or sliced
1/2 pound Monterey Jack cheese, shredded or sliced
9 thin slices Genoa salami
16 eggs
3 1/4 cups milk
1/2 cup dry white wine
4 large green onions, minced
1 tablespoon German or Dijon mustard
1/4 teaspoon pepper
1/8 teaspoon red pepper, ground
1 1/2 cup sour cream
2/3 to 1 cup Parmesan cheese

Butter 2 shallow 3-quart (9 x 13-inch) dishes. Spread bread over bottom and drizzle with butter. Sprinkle cheeses and salami over bread. Beat together eggs, milk, wine, green onion, mustard, pepper, and red pepper until foamy. Pour over cheese, salami, and bread. Cover dishes in foil, crimping edges. Refrigerate overnight or up to 24 hours. Remove from refrigerator 30 minutes before baking. Preheat oven to 325 degrees. Bake covered until set, about 1 hour. Uncover. Spread sour cream over tops and sprinkle with Parmesan cheese. Bake uncovered until crusty and brown, about 10 minutes.

Nutrient Value per Serving (makes 8 servings): 790.77 calories, 46.31g protein, 13.03g carbohydrates, 59.95g fat

Russian-Style Breast of Chicken

2 whole chicken breasts, skinned and boned
Approximately 2 ounces clarified butter
1/4 cup flour
1/8 teaspoon grated nutmeg
salt and pepper to taste

Cut chicken breasts in half. Salt and pepper lightly. Mix nutmeg with flour and dredge chicken in flour. Shake off excess flour. Melt clarified butter in heavy skillet. Quickly sauté chicken breasts until golden. Do not overcook. Remove to platter and cover with foil to keep warm. Make Paprika-Thyme Sauce according to directions below. Add chicken to sauce, including any accumulated juices. Reheat in sauce for a few minutes until warmed through.

Paprika-Thyme Sauce

1 small onion, chopped
1 tablespoon unsalted butter
2 teaspoons paprika
1 tablespoon flour
1/4 teaspoon dried thyme
1/2 cup chicken broth
1/2 cup heavy cream
juice of 1/2 lemon
salt and pepper
1 teaspoon brandy
1/4 cup sour cream

Sauté onion in butter for about 5 minutes. Add paprika, flour, thyme, and chicken broth. Simmer for 5 minutes more. Add cream, lemon juice, salt, pepper, and brandy. Cook until reduced to desired consistency. Strain sauce and set aside until ready to use. (May be prepared a day ahead of time.) Before serving, return to medium-low heat. Add sour cream, but do not let sauce boil or it will curdle.

Suggestion: Serve with Shredded Potato Cakes.

Nutrient Value per Serving (makes 4 servings): 690.81 calories, 39.90g protein, 12.62g carbohydrates, 53.52g fat

Shredded Potato Cakes

2 large baking potatoes
1/2 small onion
1 egg
1 tablespoon flour
1 tablespoon milk
salt and pepper to taste
1 tablespoon melted butter
clarified butter for sauté

Grate potatoes (using the large grating blade of a food processor works well). Grate the onion and mix with the potatoes. Place mixture in a bowl. Blend the eggs, flour, milk, and melted butter thoroughly. Salt and pepper to taste. Pour mixture over potatoes. Toss. Heat clarified butter in large, heavy skillet. Measure out approximately 1/4 cup of the potato mixture and place in skillet. Mash down to flatten. Fry until golden brown. Serve at once.

Nutrient Value per Serving (makes 2 servings): 377.26 calories, 8.57g protein, 54.57g carbohydrates, 14.41g fat

Tournedos of Beef with Shallot Sauce

beef tournedos, each 3 1/2 to 4 ounces (1 or 2 per person)
salt and freshly ground black pepper
butter and oil
1/2 cup Chablis or other dry white wine

Shallot Sauce:

1 1/2 cups Chablis
1/2 cup minced shallots
1 bay leaf
pinch of cayenne pepper
2 cups heavy cream

In a heavy saucepan (not aluminum or iron), combine all ingredients for the sauce, except the heavy cream. Boil until reduced by about two thirds. Then add the cream and cook until again reduced by about two thirds or until sauce is thick enough to coat a spoon. Set aside. Season tournedos on both sides with pepper. (You may want to tie them with string to keep their shape.) Sauté in equal amounts of oil and butter over fairly high heat until lightly browned and cooked to taste. Transfer to a warmed platter and cover with foil to keep warm. Pour off all fat and deglaze the skillet with 1/2 cup Chablis. Scrape browned bits off bottom of pan. Strain the shallots and cream sauce and add to the liquid left in the skillet (for more character, do not strain the sauce before adding it to the liquid in the skillet). Bring to a boil if sauce is not thick enough and reduce it a little more at this time. Check for seasoning. Pour a little on top of each of the tournedos and serve the rest of the sauce on the side.

Nutrient Value per Serving (makes 8 servings): 2,112.78 calories, 277.34g protein, 3.82g carbohydrates, 97.82g fat

Garnished Sauerkraut

2 pounds sauerkraut
1 large onion
1 cooking apple, cored and quartered
2 cloves garlic, chopped
fresh ground black pepper
4 juniper berries, crushed
dry white wine to cover
2 pounds Boston butt roast or pork shoulder or ribs
4 to 8 sausages (bratwurst, knockwurst, blutwurst, or a combination)
salt
oil
1 tablespoon caraway seed

Melt oil in a deep, heavy casserole. Add the onion and sauté for a few minutes until soft. Add the garlic and remove from heat. Heat oven to 300 degrees. Rinse sauerkraut and drain. Place a thick layer of sauerkraut over onions and garlic. Grind plenty of black pepper over sauerkraut. Sprinkle with half of the juniper berries and half of caraway seed. Cut pork into serving size pieces. Rub lightly with salt. Place on top of sauerkraut. Place half of the apple between meat pieces. Place rest of sauerkraut on top of meat. It should be well covered with the sauerkraut. Then sprinkle with pepper, remaining juniper berries, caraway seed, and apple pieces. Salt lightly. Add wine. Cover. Place into pre-heated oven and bake for 4 hours or longer. Before serving, sprinkle a little flour (approximately 3 tablespoons) over sauerkraut and stir. (Reduce the amount of flour if a lot of juice has cooked away.) Cover and cook on top of stove for about 10 to 15 minutes. Remove meat to a warmed platter and cover with foil to keep warm. Stir sauerkraut well to blend onions and other ingredients. Cook sausages according to package directions. Place sauerkraut on a large platter. Surround with the meat and garnish with the sausages.

Nutrient Value per Serving (makes 4 servings): 1,261.08 calories, 95.72g protein, 21.32g carbohydrates, 82.28g fat

Bread Pudding with Whiskey Sauce

1 loaf French bread
3 eggs
2 tablespoons vanilla
1 cup raisins
1 quart milk
2 cups sugar
3 tablespoons butter

Tear bread into pieces. Soak in milk and mash with hands until soft. Add rest of ingredients. Mix well. Pour into buttered baking dish and bake in 375-degree oven for 40 to 45 minutes.

Whiskey Sauce

1 stick margarine
1 cup sugar
1 egg
1/4 cup whiskey

Melt margarine. Add sugar and stir well until melted. Add 3 to 4 drops water. Beat egg slightly and temper with hot mixture. Then add rest of egg and whisk briskly so mixture will not curdle. Cool slightly and add whiskey. Serve sauce over bread pudding.

Nutrient Value per Serving (makes 6 servings): 1,334.55 calories, 28.58g protein, 233.39g carbohydrates, 33.49g fat

Apple Cake

1 cup cooking oil
2 cups sugar
3 eggs
2 1/2 cups flour
1 teaspoon baking soda
1 teaspoon baking powder
3 cups chopped apples
1 teaspoon vanilla
1 cup nuts
1 teaspoon cinnamon
1 teaspoon nutmeg

Combine oil, sugar, and eggs. Beat well. Add flour and beat thoroughly. Add remaining ingredients and stir to blend well. Grease and flour a 13 x 9-inch pan. Pour batter into pan and bake in a 350-degree oven for 1 hour.

Topping

1 cup sugar
milk
2/3 stick margarine
1 teaspoon vanilla

Place sugar in saucepan. Add just enough milk to dissolve sugar. Add remaining ingredients. Bring to a boil until a soft ball forms in ice water. Pour on cake while warm.

Nutrient Value per Serving (makes 8 servings): 835.03 calories, 6.22g protein, 102.06g carbohydrates, 46.96g fat

Prune Cake

2 cups flour
1 teaspoon baking soda
1/2 teaspoon salt
1 teaspoon cinnamon
1 teaspoon nutmeg
1 teaspoon allspice
2 1/2 cups sugar
1 cup cooking oil
2 eggs
1 teaspoon vanilla
1 cup buttermilk
1 cup cooked prunes, chopped and unsweetened
1 cup chopped nuts

Sift flour, soda, salt, and all of the spices. Cream oil, sugar, eggs, and vanilla. Add dry mixture and buttermilk alternately to creamed mixture. Mix well. Add prunes and nuts. Grease and flour a 9 x 12-inch pan. Pour batter into pan and bake in 325-degree oven for just over an hour.

Topping

1 cup sugar
2/3 stick margarine
milk
1 teaspoon vanilla

Place sugar in saucepan. Add just enough milk to dissolve sugar. Add remaining ingredients. Bring to a boil. Cook until a soft ball forms in ice water. Pour over warm cake.

Nutrient Value per Serving (makes 8 servings): 823.0 calories, 7.51g protein, 98.27g carbohydrates, 46.61g fat

Banana Nut Bread

1 cup sugar
1/2 cup shortening
1 egg
2 cups flour
1 teaspoon baking soda
1/2 teaspoon salt
1 teaspoon vanilla
1/2 cup chopped nuts
2 large or 3 small bananas, extra ripe

Cream sugar, shortening, and egg. Sift baking soda and salt into flour. Add mashed bananas and flour alternately to shortening mixture. Stir in vanilla and nuts. Bake in loaf pan in 350-degree oven for approximately 45 to 50 minutes or until a toothpick inserted in the middle comes out clean. Remove from pan and cool on a rack.

Nutrient Value per Serving (makes 4 servings): 924.93 calories, 10.99g protein, 127.72g carbohydrates, 46.15g fat

Traditional White Bread

2 packages active dry yeast
1/2 cup warm water
1 3/4 cups warm water
3 tablespoons sugar
1 tablespoon salt
2 tablespoons shortening
6 to 7 cups bread flour
butter or margarine softened

Dissolve yeast in 1/2 cup warm water in large mixing bowl. Sprinkle sugar over yeast. Stir in 1 3/4 cups warm water, salt, shortening, and 3 1/2 cups of the flour. Beat until smooth. Stir in enough remaining flour to make dough easy to handle. Turn dough out onto lightly floured surface. Knead until smooth and elastic, about 10 minutes. Place in greased bowl; turn greased side up. Cover and let rise in warm place until double, about 1 hour. Punch down dough and divide in half. Flatten each half and shape into loaves. Place loaves seam sides down in 2 greased loaf pans. Brush lightly with butter. Let rise until double, about 1 hour. Heat oven to 425 degrees. Place loaves on low rack so that tops of pans are in center of oven. Pans should not touch each other or sides of oven. Bake until loaves are deep golden brown and sound hollow when tapped, 25 to 30 minutes. Remove loaves from pans to a wire rack. Brush with butter and allow to cool.

Nutrient Value per Serving (makes 8 servings): 500.12 calories, 12.0g protein, 88.88g carbohydrates, 9.99g fat

Apple Coffee Cake

2 tablespoons shortening
1 cup sugar
1 egg
1 teaspoon vanilla
2 cups self-rising flour
1 cup milk
2 large apples

Pare, core, and slice apples. Beat remaining ingredients until smooth and blended. Pour batter into greased and floured 9-inch cake pan. Arrange apple slices on top of batter. Top with crumb mixture (see below). Bake in 375-degree oven for 35 minutes or until done.

Crumb Mixture

2/3 cup sugar
1 tablespoon flour

Combine ingredients until blended.

Nutrient Value per Serving (makes 6 servings): 464.77 calories, 6.75g protein, 96.51g carbohydrates, 6.47g fat

Ice Box Rolls

1 package dry yeast
1/2 cup sugar
2 cups warm water
1 teaspoon salt
3 tablespoons melted shortening
6 to 7 cups flour

Mix yeast with sugar and water. Allow to stand until bubbly (about 15 minutes). Stir in salt, shortening, and enough flour to make a soft dough. Turn dough out onto a floured board. Knead until smooth and satiny. Place kneaded dough in a greased bowl, cover lightly, and let rise in warm place until doubled in bulk (about 1 hour). Punch down. Cover tightly and refrigerate. Approximately 2 hours before baking, remove from refrigerator and make into rolls by pinching off pieces of dough the size of walnuts. Roll pieces in melted shortening and place in a greased baking dish with the rolls touching. Let rise in a warm place for 1 to 1 1/2 hours until doubled in size. Bake in 350-degree oven until brown (about 20 minutes).

Note: Dough may be stored in refrigerator for up to 1 week and used as needed.

Nutrient Value per Serving (makes 4 servings): 983.20 calories, 23.21g protein, 192.57g carbohydrates, 11.84 g fat

Butterscotch Pie

1 cup brown sugar
2 1/2 tablespoons flour
1/4 cup butter
1/8 teaspoon salt
1 cup scalded milk
2 egg yolks
1/2 teaspoon vanilla

Combine brown sugar, flour, butter, and salt in double boiler. Stirring constantly, cook until well blended. Add scalded milk. Remove from heat. Beat egg yolks until light. Temper beaten yolks with a little of the milk mixture. Add tempered yolks to milk mixture. Blend well and return to heat. Stirring constantly, cook until thickened. Remove from heat. Cool. Add vanilla. Pour into baked pie crust. Top with meringue (see recipe below). Bake in 300-degree oven 15 to 20 minutes to brown peaks of meringue.

Meringue

2 egg whites
1/2 teaspoon vanilla
1/4 teaspoon cream of tartar
4 tablespoons sugar

Beat egg whites with vanilla and cream of tartar at low speed to blend. Increase speed gradually to high and beat until soft peaks form. Gradually add sugar and continue beating until stiff peaks form and sugar is dissolved. Spread meringue over filling, creating peaks with back of spoon, and bake to brown peaks.

Nutrient Value per Serving (makes 8 servings): 221.17 calories, 2.89g protein, 36.49g carbohydrates, 7.62g fat

Chocolate Fudge

2 sticks margarine
5 cups sugar
2 small or 1 large package chocolate chips
1 teaspoon vanilla
1 large can Carnation evaporated milk
3 tablespoons marshmallow creme
1 tablespoon peanut butter

Over low heat, bring sugar, milk, and butter to boil in a heavy saucepan. Cook 9 minutes, stirring constantly. Remove from heat. Add chocolate chips and marshmallow creme. Let cool. Add vanilla. Beat until thick. Add peanut butter. Pour into a buttered 13x9-inch dish and refrigerate. Once completely cooled and set, cut into pieces.

Variation: Add 1 cup chopped nuts along with peanut butter.

Nutrient Value per Serving (makes 6 servings): 1,520.03 calories, 10.0g protein, 231.52g carbohydrates, 70.79g fat

Peanut Butter Fudge

2 cups sugar
1/4 cup peanut butter
1/2 cup milk
1/3 cup light corn syrup
pinch of salt
2 teaspoons butter
1 teaspoon vanilla

Mix sugar, peanut butter, milk, corn syrup, and salt in heavy saucepan. Stir well. Cook over medium heat, stirring constantly, until candy forms a soft ball in cold water. Remove from heat. Add butter. Cool fudge and add vanilla. Beat until thick. Pour into a buttered 9x9-inch dish and refrigerate. Once completely cooled and set, cut into pieces.

Nutrient Value per Serving (makes 4 servings): 577.70 calories, 4.98g protein, 121.33g carbohydrates, 10.51g fat

Cherry Cobbler

1 cup self-rising flour
1 cup sugar
1 cup milk
1 stick butter
1 can tart red cherries, pitted

Melt butter in baking dish. Mix flour, sugar, and milk together. Pour batter into melted butter. Let cool for 1 minute. Add cherries with juice; do not stir. Bake 20 minutes in 450-degree oven.

Variation: Substitute other fruits at will. Serve warm and top with vanilla ice cream.

Nutrient Value per Serving (makes 6 servings): 385.93 calories, 4.04g protein, 57.0g carbohydrates, 16.71g fat

Rice Pudding

3 eggs
2 cups milk
3/4 cup sugar
2 tablespoons melted butter
1/4 teaspoon nutmeg
2 cups cooked white rice
1 cup raisins
1/2 cup nuts (optional)

Combine eggs and milk. Beat well. Stir in remaining ingredients and turn into buttered casserole dish. Place casserole dish in pan containing about one inch hot water. Bake for 1 hour in 350-degree oven.

Nutrient Value per Serving (makes 4 servings): 592.19 calories, 12.75g protein, 92.50g carbohydrates, 21.29g fat

Chocolate Pie

2 tablespoons cornstarch
6 tablespoons sugar
2 cups milk
4 tablespoons cocoa
2 eggs, separated
1 teaspoon vanilla

Mix cornstarch, cocoa, sugar, egg yolks, and milk in heavy saucepan. Stirring constantly, boil until thickened. Remove from heat and cool slightly. Add vanilla. Pour into 8-inch baked pie shell. Beat egg whites with 2 tablespoons sugar until stiff. Spread over pie, create peaks with back of spoon, and brown in 375-degree oven.

Nutrient Value per Serving (makes 4 servings): 422.84 calories, 9.96g protein, 49.81g carbohydrates, 20.36g fat

Strawberry Pie

1 quart strawberries
1 cup sugar
1 cup water
4 tablespoons cornstarch
1/2 teaspoon red food coloring
3 tablespoons lemon juice
dash salt

Cap berries and drain. Mix remaining ingredients in heavy saucepan and cook until thick and clear. Let cool. Arrange berries in baked 9-inch pie crust. Pour cooled mixture over berries. Refrigerate.

Nutrient Value per Serving (makes 6 servings): 339.19 calories, 2.48g protein, 59.98g carbohydrates, 10.71g fat

Pineapple Coconut Cake

1 box yellow cake mix
6 ounces crushed pineapple
7-ounce package shredded coconut

Bake cake according to package directions. Cool. Drain pineapple, reserving juice for frosting.

Butter Cream Frosting

1 pound powdered sugar
1/2 cup margarine
1/8 teaspoon salt
1 teaspoon vanilla
3 to 4 tablespoons pineapple juice (substituted for milk)

Cream 1/3 cup sugar with salt and butter. Blend vanilla, 2 tablespoons juice, and remaining sugar into mixture. Add remaining juice as needed. Add some of pineapple to frosting.

Frost bottom layer of cake. Spread pineapple on top of this layer. Place second layer on top of pineapple and frost top and sides of cake. Pat coconut on top and sides over frosting.

Nutrient Value per Serving (makes 8 servings): 488.92 calories, 1.45g protein, 76.84g carbohydrates, 21.10g fat

Banana Pudding

1 recipe custard (see page 15)
3 large bananas
Vanilla Wafers

Prepare custard according to recipe directions and cool. In a 2-quart casserole dish, layer Vanilla Wafers, banana slices, and custard. Repeat for two more layers. Top with meringue (see recipe below). Bake in 300-degree oven 15 to 20 minutes to brown peaks of meringue.

Meringue

3 egg whites
1/2 teaspoon vanilla
1/4 teaspoon cream of tartar
6 tablespoons sugar

Beat egg whites with vanilla and cream of tartar at low speed to blend. Increase speed gradually to high and beat until soft peaks form. Gradually add sugar and continue beating until stiff peaks form and sugar is dissolved. Spread meringue over filling, creating peaks with back of spoon, and bake to brown peaks.

Nutrient Value per Serving (makes 4 servings): 640.17 calories, 73.26g protein, 122.98g carbohydrates, 12.72g fat

Coconut Pie

1 9-inch pie crust
1 recipe custard (see page 15)
1 16-ounce package shredded coconut

Brown pie crust according to instructions. Prepare custard according to recipe instructions and cool. Reserve 2 tablespoons coconut. Mix remaining coconut with custard and spoon into browned crust. Top with meringue (see recipe below). Sprinkle reserved coconut over meringue. Bake in 300-degree oven 15 to 20 minutes to brown coconut and peaks of meringue.

Meringue

3 egg whites
1/2 teaspoon vanilla
1/4 teaspoon cream of tartar
6 tablespoons sugar

Beat egg whites with vanilla and cream of tartar at low speed to blend. Increase speed gradually to high and beat until soft peaks form. Gradually add sugar and continue beating until stiff peaks form and sugar is dissolved. Spread meringue over filling, creating peaks with back of spoon, and bake to brown peaks.

Nutrient Value per Serving (makes 8 servings): 588.87 calories, 7.37g protein, 45.69g carbohydrates, 29.14g fat

Notes

Glossary

al dente: Firm to the bite.

blend: To mix or fuse thoroughly so that the parts are no longer separate and distinct; to mix or mingle so as to produce a desired texture or consistency.

calorie: A unit for measuring the energy produced by food when oxidized in the body.

carbohydrate: One of three classes of nutrients that supply calories to the body. Carbohydrates are a basic source of energy. They are stored in virtually all body tissues, but primarily in the liver and muscles.

chiffonnade: Leaves of Belgian endive, lettuce, or sorrel cut into shreds or strips to be used as a garnish. The chiffonnade may be used raw or braised in butter.

cholesterol: A sterol found widely in animal fats, blood, nerve tissue, and bile. Cholesterol serves as a precursor of various steroid hormones. An elevated level of blood cholesterol constitutes an increased risk of coronary heart disease.

clarified butter: Clarifying butter is intended to remove the milky fat part (to make it clear). Heat butter gently at a low temperature in a small saucepan until the butter melts and separates. Skim off the clear portion and reserve. Discard the milky sediment. Clarified butter is used for sautéing at high temperatures.

diet: Liquid and solid foods consumed regularly.
   A prescribed allowance or selection of food selected for a particular state of health or disease.

dredge: To coat or sprinkle with flour, cornmeal, or something similar.

fat: Adipose tissue of the body.

Any of various mixtures of semisolid or solid triglycerides found in adipose tissue of animals or in the seeds of plants.

fold: To gently blend one mixture into another. Typically, a rubber spatula is inserted at the outer edge of the bowl; the bowl is rotated slightly while bringing the spatula up through the mixture. Continue until both mixtures are incorporated.

fortify: Add additional nutrients to food.

lactose: A sugar found in milk.

mineral: An inorganic element or compound required by the body. Minerals are essential components of all cells. Examples include calcium, phosphorus, sodium, copper, iodine, magnesium, iron, and potassium.

nutrient: The part of foodstuffs that supply the body with elements needed for metabolism. Required nutrients include carbohydrates, fats, proteins, minerals, vitamins, water, and electrolytes.

pare: To trim, shave, or remove an outside part (as the skin of an apple).

protein: Any of a large class of complex nitrogenous substances occurring naturally in plants and animals. Proteins yield amino acids when broken down in water and are essential for the growth and repair of human tissue.

shallot: A small onion whose clustered bulbs are used for flavoring. Shallots are similar to garlic, but milder in flavor.

sugar: Any of a class of sweet, crystalline, soluble carbohydrates belonging to the monosaccharose and disaccharose groups.

temper: To bring to the proper consistency or texture by mixing with something or treating in some way.

vitamin: Any of a number of organic substances other than carbohydrates, fats, minerals, organic salts, or proteins essential for regulation of body metabolism, growth, and development.

whisk: A utensil consisting of wire loops fixed in a handle, for whipping egg whites, cream, etc.

To whip (egg whites, cream, etc.).

Index by Food Groups
and Recipe Types

Baked apples, 54
Baked onions, 44
Baked stuffed tomatoes, 75
Black beans, 39
Brussels sprouts and artichokes,
　52
Cabbage stew, 51
Fried apples, 44
Marinated cucumbers, 43
Peas with Boston lettuce, 45
Peas paysanne, 50
Red beans, 55
Roasted potatoes, 48
Sautéed cocktail tomatoes, 24
Sautéed cocktail tomatoes
　　　and snow peas, 49
Shredded potato cakes, 51,82
Steamed carrots, 25
Stewed tomatoes, 45

MEAT

Beef stew, 71
Tournedos of beef with shallot
　　sauce, 83

POULTRY

Bacon-wrapped chicken breasts, 25
Chicken breasts with grapes, 28
Chicken piccate, 26
Russian-style breast of chicken, 81

RICE, PASTAS, AND DUMPLINGS

Baked egg noodles, 62
Curried rice, 33
Dumplings, 63
Garlic pasta, 68
German potato dumplings, 65
Rice with leeks, 46
White rice, 32

SALADS

Cottage cheese Jello salad, 14
Four-bean salad, 43
German potato salad, 46
Lime Jello salad, 14
Orange Jello salad, 14
Pasta salad, 58
Spinach and grapefruit salad, 49
24-hour fruit salad, 47

SOUPS

Bean soup, 38
Broccoli and cheese soup, 60
Cheese soup, 16
Cream of carrot soup, 17
Cream of tomato soup, 37
Creamy chicken noodle soup, 59
Creamy potato soup, 61
Creamy pumpkin soup, 18
Easy egg drop soup, 13
Easy tortellini soup, 59
French onion soup, 76
Watercress soup, 63

Alphabetical Index

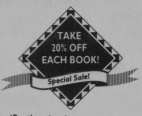

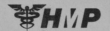

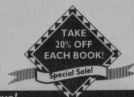